KETO DIET PIZZA & PASTA
Cookbook for Beginners

Foolproof Recipes
for Busy People on Keto Diet

Valentina Arcuri

© Copyright 2019 - Valentina Arcuri - All rights reserved.

ISBN: 978-1676907305

Legal Notice:

This book is copyright protected. This is only for personal use. You cannot amend, distribute, sell, use, quote or paraphrase any part or the content within this book without the consent of the author or copyright owner. Legal action will be pursued if this is breached.

The information provided herein is stated to be truthful and consistent, in that any liability, regarding inattention or otherwise, by any usage or abuse of any policies, processes, or directions contained within is the solitary and complete responsibility of the recipient reader. Under no circumstances will any legal liability or blame be held against the publisher for any reparation, damages, or monetary loss due to the information herein, either directly or indirectly.

CONTENTS

INTRODUCTION 5
THE KETOGENIC DIET 6
ANTIPASTI 8
Blackberry Prosciutto Appetizer 8
Italian Meatballs 9
Caramelized Onion Dip 10
Stuffed Mushrooms 11
Italian Roasted Turnip Bites 12
Tomato-Basil Bruschetta 13
Antipasti Kabobs 14
Beef Carpaccio 15
Avocado-Chimichurri Appetizer 16
Caprese Salad Stacks with Pesto & Anchovies 17

PASTA 18
Parsley-Lime Shrimp Pasta 18
Coconut Tuna Zucchini Bake 19
Creamy Garlic Shrimp with Angel Hair Shirataki 20
Creamy Salmon Shirataki Fettucine 21
Creamy Mussel with Shirataki 22
Beef Alfredo Squash Spaghetti 23
Beef-Asparagus Shirataki Mix 24
Garlic-Butter Steak Bites with Shirataki Fettuccine 25
Keto Pasta with Mediterranean Meatballs 26
Thai Beef Shirataki Stir-Fry 28
Beef Ragu with Veggie Pasta 29
Classic Beef Lasagna 30
Creamy Sun-Dried & Parsnip Noodles 31
Keto Beef Carbonara 32
Pesto Parmesan Pork with Green Pasta 33
Pork Lo Mein 34
Pasta & Cheese Pulled Pork 36
Creamy Pork with Green Beans and Keto Fettuccine 38
Delicious Sambal Pork Noodles 39
Lemongrass Pork with Spaghetti Squash 40
Pork Avocado Keto Noodles 41
Chinese Pork and Celeriac Noodles 42
Garlic Pecorino Kohlrabi with Sausage 43
Chicken Alfredo Zoodles 44
One-Pot Spicy Cheddar Pasta 45

Creamy Tuscan Chicken Linguine 46
Tomato Kale Chicken Skillet with Keto Linguine 48
Cajun Chicken Fettuccine 50
Saffron Chicken and Pasta 52
Mustard Chicken Shirataki 54
Creamy Mushrooms with Broccoli Pasta 55
Cauliflower Casserole with Shirataki 56
Tofu Spaghetti Bolognese 57
Balsamic Veggie-Pasta Mix 58
Vegetarian Fajita Pasta 60
Roasted Vegetable Spaghetti 61
Spicy Veggie Pasta Bake 62
Super Green Pasta Skillet 64
Broccoli and Pepper Spaghetti 65
Veggie Pasta Primavera 66

PIZZA 67

Pepperoni Fat Head Pizza 67
BBQ Beef Pizza 68
Chicken-Basil Pizza 69
Chicken Bacon Ranch Pizza 70
Kale-Artichoke Pizza 71
Sausage-Pepper Pizza 72
Tomato-Prosciutto Pizza 73
Vegetarian Spinach-Olive Pizza 74
Cauliflower-Pepperoni Pizza Casserole 75
Italian Mushroom Pizza 76
Extra Cheesy Pizza 77
Spicy and Smoky Pizza 78
Taco pizza 79
Broccoli-Pepper Pizza 80
Caramelized Onion and Goat Cheese Pizza 81
Shrimp Scampi Pizza 82
Strawberry-Tomato Pizza 83
Mediterranean Pizza 84
Pesto Arugula Pizza 85
Four Cheese Mexican Pizza 86

SOMETHING SWEET 87

Italian Raspberry-Coconut Cake 87
Balsamic Strawberry Ricotta 88
Blueberry Sorbet 88
Strawberry Mousse 89
Sweet Lemon Panna Cotta 90

INTRODUCTION

Understanding the craze of the Ketogenic Diet

I'll tell you. Long before we got all "richly" about meals – I mean loading our plates with meats, cheeses, and creamy goodness; the folks dating back from 500 BC were already on this spree.

To them, they left carbohydrates out of their diets to treat epilepsy in children and ate foods with high fats, proteins, and many green vegetables. And guess what? It worked!

This is what the Ketogenic Diet is, removing high carbs from foods and eating high fats and proteins instead. It solves a diverse range of ailments by merely reducing the amounts of sugars in the body and allowing good fats play a healing role.

Usually, the body will "lazily" burn energy from carbohydrates because it is easiest while fats, which are supposed to be burned for energy, sit in the body and do nothing. Because they lay idle, your love handles keep increasing, your cheeks get plumper, and you find fats in all the areas of your body that you will rather prefer that they weren't.

Thanks to the many researchers that dug out this ancient secret, it is a diet for now and for the future. Having been embraced by many medical practitioners and healthy living enthusiasts, it is of no surprise that the Ketogenic Diet is one of the first recommendations for curing varying ailments – this is how far good craze has gone.

For me, it is a feel-good kind of a diet. It keeps me sane, light-weighted, and feeling fresh within and out; I couldn't ask for more. As a big lover of Italian food and most particularly, pasta and pizza, I was extremely unhappy not to be able to eat my favorite dishes, which turn out to be full of carbs. So I decided to roll up my sleaves and get to work - pizza can't be something bad for you if made healthy.

In this book, I present you with effortless and tasty Keto options for our most beloved dishes. I hope you'd explore what works best for you and enjoy an easier adaptation to this new keto lifestyle.

THE KETOGENIC DIET

The positives of the Ketogenic Diet

Blood Sugar Control

Starchy foods and sugary foods produce sugars in the body. This is why people with diabetes suffer, and to my surprise, in the past, meal plans created for people with diabetes were loaded with carbohydrates, fruits, and processed milk. So wrong!

By avoiding carbohydrates, the amount of sugars in the body drops drastically, which requires a relative reduction in the use of diabetic medication.

Significant enough, there are many testimonies of the Keto diet healing diabetics completely; that's some good news right there!

Weight loss

It goes without stressing that you're up for a significant weight shed once you start dieting the Keto way. Why so? Because your body now burns all the stored up fat in your body for energy.

Like I said earlier when on carbs, the body's duty to consume fats gets dormant and will rather burn carbs. But, when carbohydrates are reduced, the body is moved into a metabolic state called ketosis where it is forced to burn fats.

Appetite Control

Ever wondered why there is a word as "sweet-tooth"? The more sugars you eat, the more of it you will want. Therefore, the unexpected hunger pangs after taking sugary foods or fruits.

Appetite levels increase, not necessarily, because the body needs food. It is because the body burns sugars fast and creates a false alert that it needs more food. The truth is it just needs some SUGAR.

On the keto diet, fat burns slower keeping the body fuller for an extended period. I usually find myself eating twice a day on a healthy meal because my breakfast is fat-rich and keeps me full past my lunch period sometimes. If hungry in between meals, I snack on a Keto option, and I'm good.

Energy Levels

Starch and sugars are tricky – they satisfy fast, but burn out fast. When this happens, the body is left weak and craves more carbs only to be burned quickly again. Energy levels then fluctuate causing most parts of the body to be less vibrant.

On the other hand, feeding on high fats and Proteins create a steady level of energy because fats and Protein burn gradually and in a consistent manner.

Keto Diet and Insulin Resistance

On a high carb diet, the body breaks starch into useful sugar components known as glucose, which is transported to the muscles and tissues as energy. The carrier of this glucose is insulin – meant to be a good thing.

However, in cases where the body becomes resistant to insulin, sugar breaks lose in the body. Once, the liver, cells in the muscles, and fats stop absorbing the sugars, they find their way into the blood and have a free flow – diabetes sets in.

Through the Keto diet, this problem is prevented because the body is naturally reduced of sugars through carb reduction hence there is more control over the amount of sugar needed in the body.

Why Fat and Proteins – does this mean carbohydrates are bad?

No, don't get it twisted. Carbohydrates aren't bad for the sense that they are nature's gift for feeding. However, for their starchy and sugary components, a small measure of carb intake should be considered to avoid increased sugar levels and low energy.

Fats and proteins, on the other hand, are safer options to consume in larger quantities. They are a more sustainable way of providing energy to the body, lead to weight loss, and are entirely healthy to the body.

Meanwhile, fats can be categorized into two parts: good and bad fats. Below I give examples of some good fats, but mostly these are sourced from natural ingredients like meat, fatty fish, nuts, avocados, tofu, and seeds. While bad fats are often processed products, for example, some "vegetable oils."

Concisely, you want to ensure that you are deriving your fats from natural sources and using vegetables with low carb counts if you need to eat carbohydrates like rice.

ANTIPASTI

Blackberry Prosciutto Appetizer

A fantastic way to blend fruit with meat for starters. Warm a party with these!

Total Time: 24 minutes | **Serving**: 4

Ingredients

4 zero bread slices
¾ cup organic balsamic vinegar
2 tbsp erythritol
1 cup fresh blackberries
2 garlic cloves, minced
1 cup crumbled goat cheese
¼ tsp dry Italian seasoning
1 tbsp almond milk
4 thin prosciutto slices

Directions

Cut the bread into 3 pieces each and arrange on a baking sheet. Place under the broiler and toast for 1 to 2 minutes on each side or until golden brown. Remove from the oven and set aside.

In a small saucepan, add the balsamic vinegar and stir in the erythritol until dissolved. Boil the mixture over medium heat until reduced to half of a cup, 5 minutes.

Turn the heat off and carefully stir in the blackberries making sure that they do not break open. Set aside.

In a blender, add the garlic, goat cheese, Italian seasoning and almond milk. Process until smooth.

Brush one side of the toasted bread with the balsamic reduction and top with the cheese mixture. Cut each prosciutto slice into 3 pieces and place on the bread. Top with some of the whole blackberries from the balsamic mixture. Serve immediately.

Nutritional info per serving:

Calories 175; Fats 7g; Net Carbs 8.7g; Protein 18.5g

Italian Meatballs

Meatballs are pleasing for different servings and ideal for starters.

Total Time: 1 hour 30 minutes | **Serving**: 4

Ingredients

½ lb ground beef
½ lb ground sweet Italian sausage
¾ cup pork rinds
½ cup finely grated Parmesan cheese
2 eggs
1 tsp onion powder
1 tsp garlic powder
1 tbsp chopped fresh basil
Salt and black pepper to taste
2 tsp dried Italian seasoning
3 tbsp olive oil + extra for greasing
2 ½ cups unsweetened marinara sauce
Mini bamboo skewers

Directions

In a large bowl, add the beef, Italian sausage, pork rinds, Parmesan cheese, eggs, onion powder, garlic powder, basil, salt, black pepper, and Italian seasoning. Grease your hands with some olive oil and form 1-inch meatballs out of the mixture.

Heat the remaining olive oil in a large skillet and working in batches, brown the meatballs on all sides, about 15 minutes.

Pour the marinara sauce into a large pot and arrange the meatballs in the sauce in a single layer; spoon some of the sauce over the meatballs to coat. Close the lid and cook over low heat for 45 minutes to 1 hour or until the meatballs are cooked within.

Using a spoon, remove the meatballs onto a serving platter and insert the skewers.

Serve immediately.

Nutritional info per serving:

Calories 513; Fats 24.5g; Net Carbs 20.4g Protein 35.7g

Caramelized Onion Dip

Onions? You needn't worry about the intense flavor of onions here as these work well into the cream mixture with some natural sweetness.

Total Time: 30 minutes | **Serving**: 4

Ingredients

2 tbsp butter
3 medium yellow onions, thinly sliced
1 tsp swerve sugar
1 tsp salt
¼ cup white wine
2 cups sour cream
8 oz cream cheese, room temperature
2 tbsp chopped fresh parsley
½ tbsp Worcestershire sauce

Directions

Melt the butter in a skillet over medium heat.

Add the onions, swerve sugar, and salt, cook with frequent stirring for 10 to 15 minutes.

Add a quarter of the white wine, stir and allow sizzling out. Repeat adding and cooking the white wine in the same manner until exhausted. The onions should be golden brown by now, 10 minutes.

Turn the heat off and use kitchen scissors to snip the onions into little bits.

In a serving bowl, mix the sour cream and cream cheese until well combined.

Add the onions, parsley, and Worcestershire sauce; stir well into the cream.

Taste the dip and adjust the seasoning with salt.

Serve immediately with celery sticks.

Nutritional info per serving:

Calories 383; Fats 34.1g; Net Carbs 8.3g Protein 8.3g

Stuffed Mushrooms

Who wouldn't grab a bite of stuffed mushrooms? They are always perfect for starting a party.

Total Time: 30 minutes | **Serving**: 4

Ingredients

¼ cup pork rinds
½ cup grated Pecorino Romano cheese
2 garlic cloves, minced
1 tbsp chopped fresh mint leaves
2 tbsp chopped fresh parsley
Salt and black pepper to taste
¼ cup ground walnuts
1/3 cup olive oil
12 large white button mushrooms, stemmed

Directions

Preheat the oven to 400 F.

In a medium bowl, mix the pork rinds, Pecorino Romano cheese, garlic, mint leaves, parsley, salt, and black pepper.

Brush a baking sheet with 2 tablespoons of the olive oil. Spoon the cheese mixture into the mushrooms and arrange on the baking sheet. Top with the ground walnuts and drizzle the remaining olive oil on the mushrooms.

Bake in the oven for 20 minutes or until the mushrooms are tender and the top is golden.

Transfer the mushrooms to a serving platter and serve afterwards.

Nutritional info per serving:

Calories 292; Fats 25.2g; Net Carbs 7.1g Protein 7.7g

Italian Roasted Turnip Bites

These may serve as a snack too, they are cheesy with a tasty crunch to them.

Total Time: 1 hour | **Serving**: 4

Ingredients

1 lb turnips
½ cup olive oil
2 garlic cloves, minced
1 tbsp chopped fresh parsley + extra for garnishing
2 tbsp chopped fresh oregano
3 tbsp dried Italian seasoning
¼ cup unsweetened marinara sauce
¼ cup finely grated mozzarella cheese

Directions

Preheat the oven to 400 F and grease a baking sheet with cooking spray. Set aside.

Peel the turnips and slice into 1-inch rounds. Pour the slices into a large bowl and toss well with the olive oil.

Add the garlic, parsley, oregano, and Italian seasoning, and mix well.

Arrange the turnips on the baking sheet in a single layer and roast for 25 minutes, flipping halfway, until softened.

Next, remove from the oven and brush the marinara sauce on top. Sprinkle the mozzarella cheese on the turnips. Bake in the oven until the cheese is golden, 15 minutes.

Garnish with parsley and serve warm.

Nutritional info per serving:

Calories 326; Fats 28.8g; Net Carbs 3.8g; Protein 4.8g

Tomato-Basil Bruschetta

An impressive way to kick off any meal. Bright red tomatoes with fresh basil make for an excellent look and aroma.

Total Time: 1 hour 15 minutes | **Serving**: 4

Ingredients

3 ripe tomatoes, chopped
6 fresh basil leaves
5 tbsp olive oil + extra for topping
Salt to taste
4 slices zero carb bread
1 garlic clove, halved

Directions

In a medium bowl, mix the tomatoes and basil until adequately combined.

Drizzle with 2 tablespoons of olive oil and salt but do not stir. Set aside uncovered to marinate for 45 minutes to 1 hour.

Almost when the marinating time is over, cut the bread slices into halves. Brush with the remaining olive oil, arrange on a baking sheet and place under the oven's broiler. Cook for 1 to 2 minutes on each side or until toasted and light brown.

Transfer the bread to a plate and gently rub the garlic on both sides of the slices.

Mix the tomato topping and spoon onto the bread slices.

Drizzle a little more of olive oil on top and serve.

Nutritional info per serving:

Calories 212; Fats 19.1g; Net Carbs 2.7g; Protein 7.9g

Antipasti Kabobs

When not in the mood for a full antipasti platter, these mini kabobs will save some time and will go around nicely.

Total Time: 45 minutes | **Serving**: 4

Ingredients
1 zucchini
8 cubes cheddar cheese
4 mini bamboo skewers
8 cherry tomatoes
8 fresh mint leaves
Salt to taste

Directions
Using a mandolin cutter, shred four thin, long slices of the zucchini.

Lay the zucchini slices on a flat surface and place two cheddar cubes on one end of each slice. Make sure that they are closely placed. Wrap the zucchini around the cheese cubes and insert a skewer each to secure.

Alternately, thread the tomatoes and mint leaves onto the skewers and season with salt.

Place the skewers on a plate, cover with plastic wrap, and chill for 30 minutes.

Serve afterwards.

Nutritional info per serving:
Calories 93; Fats 3.9g; Net Carbs 1.78g; Protein 6.8g

Beef Carpaccio

Mimicking a salad but keeping things simple to create more space in the tummy for the main course.

Total Time: 10 minutes | **Serving**: 4

Ingredients

1 tbsp olive oil
½ lemon, juiced
Salt and black pepper to taste
¼ lb rare roast beef, very thinly sliced
1 ½ cups baby arugula
¼ cup finely grated Parmesan cheese

Directions

In a small bowl, whisk the olive oil, lemon juice, salt, and black pepper until well combined.

Spread the beef on a large serving plate, top with the arugula and drizzle the olive oil mixture on top. Add the Parmesan cheese.

Serve immediately.

Nutritional info per serving:

Calories 106; Fats 4.8g; Net Carbs 4.12g; Protein 10.4g

Avocado-Chimichurri Appetizer

A better way to use avocados while combining them with chimichurri on pieces of low carb bread.

Total Time: 15 minutes | **Serving**: 4

Ingredients

4 slices zero carb bread
¼ cup + 2 tbsp olive oil
2 tbsp red wine vinegar
1 lemon, juiced
Salt and black pepper to taste
3 garlic cloves, minced
½ tsp red chili flakes
½ tsp dried oregano
½ cup chopped fresh parsley
2 avocados, pitted, peeled and cubed

Directions

Cut the bread slices in half, brush both sides with 2 tbsp of the olive oil, and arrange on a baking sheet. Place under the broiler and toast for 1 to 2 minutes per side or until golden brown. Remove from the oven and set aside.

In a medium bowl, mix the remaining olive oil, red wine vinegar, lemon juice, salt, black pepper, garlic, and red chili flakes. Stir in the oregano and parsley.

Fold in the avocados until well coated.

Spoon the mixture onto the bread slices and serve immediately.

Nutritional info per serving:

Calories 300; Fats 26.6g; Net Carbs 9.6g; Protein 9.1g

Caprese Salad Stacks with Pesto & Anchovies

Easy! Instead of a Caprese salad plate, stack the ingredients one on another. Also, don't miss out on the pesto feature.

Total Time: 10 minutes | **Serving**: 4

Ingredients
2 large red tomatoes, cut into 3 slices
12 (1-inch each) fresh mozzarella cheese slices
2 large yellow tomatoes, cut into 3 slices
1 cup basil pesto, olive oil-based
4 anchovy fillets in oil

Directions
On a serving platter, alternately stack one red tomato, one mozzarella cheese, one yellow tomato, one mozzarella slice, one red tomato slice, and then one mozzarella cheese. Repeat making 3 more stacks in the same manner.

Spoon the pesto all over the snacks making sure that they are well-covered with the pesto.

Arrange the anchovy fillets on top and serve immediately.

Nutritional info per serving:
Calories 178; Fats 9.9g; Net Carbs 3.5g Protein 17.3g

PASTA

FISH & SEAFOOD

Parsley-Lime Shrimp Pasta

A classic that never fades! Incorporating Parmesan cheese makes the dish better!

Total Time: 20 minutes | **Serving**: 4

Ingredients

2 tbsp butter
1 lb jumbo shrimp, peeled and deveined
4 garlic cloves, minced
1 pinch red chili flakes
¼ cup white wine
1 lime, zested and juiced
3 medium zucchinis, spiralized
Salt and black pepper to taste
2 tbsp chopped parsley
1 cup grated Parmesan cheese for topping

Directions

Melt the butter in a large skillet and cook the shrimp until starting to turn pink.

Flip and stir in the garlic and red chili flakes. Cook further for 1 minute or until the shrimp is pink and opaque. Transfer to a plate and set aside.

Pour the wine and lime juice into the skillet, and cook until reduced by a quarter. Meanwhile, stir to deglaze the bottom of the pot.

Mix in the zucchinis, lime zest, shrimp, and parsley. Season with salt and black pepper, and toss everything well. Cook until the zucchinis is slightly tender for 2 minutes.

Dish the food onto serving plates and top generously with the Parmesan cheese.

Nutritional info per serving:

Calories 255; Fats 8.4g; Net Carbs 9.8g; Protein 32.1g

Coconut Tuna Zucchini Bake

The flavor of coconut makes this tuna bake unique. Make sure to always include it.

Total Time: 40 minutes | **Serving**: 4

Ingredients

1 tbsp butter
1 cup green beans, chopped
1 bunch asparagus, trimmed and cut into 1-inch pieces
2 tbsp arrowroot starch
2 cups coconut milk
4 medium zucchinis, spiralized
1 cup grated Parmesan cheese
1 (15 oz) can tuna in water, drained and flaked
Salt and black pepper to taste

Directions

Preheat the oven to 380 F.

Melt the butter in a medium skillet and sauté the green beans and asparagus until softened, about 5 minutes. Set aside.

In a medium saucepan, mix the arrowroot starch with the coconut milk. Bring to a boil over medium heat with frequent stirring until thickened, 3 minutes. Stir in half of the Parmesan cheese until melted.

Mix in the green beans, asparagus, zucchinis and tuna. Season with salt and black pepper.

Transfer the mixture to a baking dish and cover the top with the remaining Parmesan cheese.

Bake in the oven until the cheese melts and golden on top, 20 minutes.

Remove the food from the oven and serve warm.

Nutritional info per serving:

Calories 389; Fats 34.2g; Net Carbs 11.1g; Protein 11.1g

Creamy Garlic Shrimp with Angel Hair Shirataki

Another way to boost up the look of your shrimp. An excellent pair for shirataki noodles.

Total Time: 25 minutes | **Serving**: 4

Ingredients

For the shrimp sauce:

- 1 tbsp olive oil
- 1 lb shrimp, peeled and deveined
- Salt and black pepper to taste
- 2 tbsp unsalted butter
- 6 garlic cloves, minced
- ½ cup dry white wine
- 1 ½ cups heavy cream
- ½ cup grated Asiago cheese
- 2 tbsp chopped fresh parsley

For the angel hair shirataki:

- 2 (8 oz) packs angel hair shirataki noodles
- Salt to season

Directions

For the shrimp sauce:

Heat the olive oil in a large skillet, season the shrimp with salt and black pepper, and cook in the oil on both sides until pink and opaque, 2 minutes. Set aside.

Melt the butter in the skillet and sauté the garlic until fragrant. Stir in the white wine and cook until reduced by half, meanwhile, scraping the bottom of the pan to deglaze.

Reduce the heat to low and stir in the heavy cream. Allow simmering for 1 minute and stir in the Asiago cheese to melt. Return the shrimp to the sauce and sprinkle the parsley on top. Adjust the taste with salt and black pepper, if needed.

For the angel hair shirataki:

Bring 2 cups of water to a boil in a pot. Strain the shirataki pasta through a colander and rinse very well under hot running water. Allow proper draining and pour the shirataki pasta into the boiling water. Take off the heat, let sit for 3 minutes and strain again.

Place a dry skillet over medium heat and stir-fry the shirataki pasta until visibly dry and makes a squeaky sound when stirred, 1 to 2 minutes. Season with salt and plate. Top the shirataki pasta with the shrimp sauce and serve warm.

Nutritional info per serving:

Calories 493; Fats 31.8g; Net Carbs 16.1g; Protein 33.7g

Creamy Salmon Shirataki Fettucine

Pairing fettuccine with salmon in a creamy sauce is always an excellent idea, and you'll appreciate the effort put into this.

Total Time: 35 minutes | **Serving**: 4

Ingredients

For the shirataki fettuccine:

2 (8 oz) packs shirataki fettuccine

For the creamy salmon sauce:

5 tbsp butter
4 salmon fillets, cut into 2-inch cubes
Salt and black pepper to taste
3 garlic cloves, minced
1 ¼ cups heavy cream
½ cup dry white wine
1 tsp grated lemon zest
1 cup baby spinach
Lemon wedges for garnishing

Directions

For the shirataki fettuccine:

Boil 2 cups of water in a pot over medium heat. Strain the shirataki pasta through a colander and rinse very well under hot running water. Pour the shirataki pasta into the boiling water. Take off the heat, let sit for 3 minutes and strain again.

Place a dry skillet over medium heat and stir-fry the shirataki pasta until visibly dry, and makes a squeaky sound when stirred, 1 to 2 minutes. Take off the heat and set aside.

For the salmon sauce:

Melt half of the butter in a large skillet; season the salmon with salt, black pepper, and cook in the butter until golden brown on all sides and flaky within, 8 minutes. Transfer to a plate and set aside. Add the remaining butter to the skillet to melt and stir in the garlic. Cook until fragrant, 1 minute.

Mix in heavy cream, white wine, lemon zest, salt, and pepper. Allow boiling over low heat for 5 minutes. Stir in spinach, allow wilting for 2 minutes and stir in shirataki fettuccine and salmon until well-coated in the sauce. Garnish with the lemon wedges.

Nutritional info per serving:

Calories 795; Fats 45.8g; Net Carbs 20.1g; Protein 72.2g

Creamy Mussel with Shirataki

I love the rich play of mussel meat and mussels in the shells in this creamy sauce. Enjoy it with your shirataki pasta!

Total Time: 25 minutes | **Serving**: 4

Ingredients

For the angel hair shirataki:

2 (8 oz) packs angel hair shirataki

For the creamy mussels:

1 lb mussels, debearded and rinsed
1 cup white wine
4 tbsp olive oil
3 shallots, finely chopped
6 garlic cloves, minced
2 tsp red chili flakes
½ cup fish stock
1 ½ cups heavy cream
2 tbsp chopped fresh parsley
Salt and black pepper to taste

Directions

For the angel hair shirataki:

Bring 2 cups of water to a boil in a pot over medium heat. Strain shirataki pasta through a colander and rinse very well under hot running water. Remove pot from the heat.

Drain and transfer the shirataki into boiling water. Take off the heat, let sit for 3 minutes and strain again. Place a large dry skillet over medium heat and stir-fry the shirataki pasta until visibly dry, 1 to 2 minutes. Take off the heat and set aside.

For the creamy mussels:

Pour mussels and white wine into a pot, cover, and cook for 4 minutes. Occasionally stir until the mussels have opened. Strain the mussels and reserve the cooking liquid. Allow cooling, discard any mussels with closed shells, and remove the meat out of ¾ of the mussel shells. Set aside with the remaining mussels in the shells.

Heat olive oil in a skillet and sauté shallots, garlic, and chili flakes for 3 minutes. Mix in reduced wine and fish stock. Allow boiling and whisk in the remaining butter and then the heavy cream. Taste the sauce and adjust the taste with salt, pepper, and mix in parsley. Pour in the shirataki pasta, mussels and toss well in the sauce. Serve afterwards.

Nutritional info per serving:

Calories 471; Fats 33.8g; Net Carbs 18.9g; Protein 18.8g

MEAT & POULTRY

BEEF

Beef Alfredo Squash Spaghetti

Instead of beef Alfredo with zoodles, I thought it would taste better with squash spaghetti. And it did!

Total Time: 1 hour and 20 minutes | **Serving**: 4

Ingredients

For the pasta:

2 medium spaghetti squashes, halved
2 tbsp olive oil

For the sauce:

2 tbsp butter
1 lb ground beef
½ tsp garlic powder
Salt and black pepper to taste
1 tsp arrowroot starch
1 ½ cups heavy cream
A pinch of nutmeg
1/3 cup finely grated Parmesan cheese
1/3 cup finely grated mozzarella cheese

Directions

Preheat the oven to 375 F and line a baking dish with foil. Set aside.

Season the squash with the olive oil, salt, and black pepper. Place the squash on the baking dish, open side up and roast for 45 to 50 minutes until the squash is tender. When ready, remove the squash from the oven, allow cooling and use two forks to shred the inner part of the noodles. Set aside.

Melt the butter in a medium pot, add the beef, garlic powder, salt, and black pepper, cook until brown, 10 minutes.

Stir in the arrowroot starch, heavy cream, and nutmeg. Cook until the sauce thickens, 2 to 3 minutes. Spoon the sauce into the squashes and cover with the Parmesan and mozzarella cheeses.

Place under the oven's broiler and cook until the cheeses melt and golden brown, 2 to 3 minutes. Remove from the oven and serve warm.

Nutritional info per serving:

Calories 563; Fats 42g; Net Carbs 4g; Protein 36.5g

Beef-Asparagus Shirataki Mix

A simple pasta mix with asparagus, yet satisfying and tasty!

Total Time: 40 minutes | **Serving**: 4

Ingredients

For the angel hair shirataki:

2 (8 oz) packs angel hair shirataki

For the beef-asparagus base:

1 lb ground beef
3 tbsp olive oil
1 lb fresh asparagus, cut into 1-inch pieces
2 large shallots, finely chopped
3 garlic cloves, minced
Salt and black pepper to taste
1 cup finely grated Parmesan cheese for topping

Directions

For the angel hair shirataki:

Bring 2 cups of water to a boil in a medium pot over medium heat. Strain the shirataki pasta through a colander and rinse very well under hot running water. Drain properly and transfer the shirataki pasta into the boiling water. Cook for 3 minutes and strain again.

Place a dry large skillet over medium heat and stir-fry the shirataki pasta until visibly dry, 1 to 2 minutes. Take off the heat and set aside.

For the beef-asparagus base:

Heat a large non-stick skillet over medium heat and add the beef. Cook while breaking the lumps that form until brown, 10 minutes. Use a slotted spoon to transfer the beef to a plate and discard the drippings.

Heat olive oil in skillet and sauté asparagus until tender, 7 minutes. Stir in shallots and garlic and cook for 2 minutes. Season with salt and pepper. Stir in the beef, shirataki and toss until well combined. Adjust the taste with salt and black pepper as desired.

Dish the food onto serving plates and garnish generously with the Parmesan cheese.

Nutritional info per serving:

Calories 513; Fats 24.7g; Net Carbs 21.4g; Protein 43.8g

Garlic-Butter Steak Bites with Shirataki Fettucine

An easy dinner fix, but infused with exciting garlic flavors!

Total Time: 30 minutes | **Serving**: 4

Ingredients

For the shirataki fettuccine:

2 (8 oz) packs shirataki fettuccine

For the garlic-butter steak bites:

4 tbsp butter
1 lb thick-cut New York strip steaks, cut into 1-inch cubes
Salt and black pepper to taste
4 garlic cloves, mined
2 tbsp chopped fresh parsley
1 cup freshly grated Pecorino Romano cheese

Directions

For the shirataki fettuccine:

Boil 2 cups of water in a medium pot over medium heat.

Strain the shirataki pasta through a colander and rinse very well under hot running water.

Allow proper draining and pour the shirataki pasta into the boiling water. Cook for 3 minutes and strain again.

Place a dry skillet over medium heat and stir-fry the shirataki pasta until visibly dry, and makes a squeaky sound when stirred, 1 to 2 minutes. Take off the heat and set aside.

For the garlic-butter steak bites:

Melt the butter in a large skillet, season the steaks with salt, black pepper and cook in the butter until brown, and cooked through, 10 minutes.

Stir in the garlic and cook until fragrant, 1 minute.

Mix in the parsley and shirataki pasta; toss well and season with salt and black pepper.

Dish the food, top with the Pecorino Romano cheese and serve immediately.

Nutritional info per serving:

Calories 422; Fats 22.4g; Net Carbs 17.3g; Protein 36.5g

Keto Pasta with Mediterranean Meatballs

The intense blend of Mediterranean flavors make this dish addictive. To trust my word, try it once and attest to this fact.

Total Time: 90 minutes + overnight chilling | **Serving**: 4

Ingredients

For the keto pasta:

1 cup shredded mozzarella cheese
1 egg yolk

For the sauce:

3 tbsp olive oil
2 yellow onions, chopped
6 garlic cloves, minced
2 tbsp unsweetened tomato paste
2 large tomatoes, chopped
¼ tsp saffron powder
2 cinnamon sticks
4 ½ cups chicken broth
Salt and black pepper to taste

For the Mediterranean meatballs:

2 cups pork rinds
1 lb ground beef
1 egg
¼ cup almond milk
6 garlic cloves, minced
Salt and black pepper to taste
½ tsp coriander powder
¼ tsp nutmeg powder
1 tbsp smoked paprika
1 ½ tsp fresh ginger paste
1 tsp cumin powder
½ tsp cayenne pepper
1 ½ tsp turmeric powder
½ tsp cloves powder
4 tbsp chopped cilantro
4 tbsp chopped scallions

4 tbsp chopped parsley
¼ cup almond flour
¼ cup olive oil
1 cup crumbled feta cheese for serving

Directions

For the pasta:

Pour the cheese into a medium safe-microwave bowl and melt in the microwave for 2 minutes while stirring at 20-second intervals until fully melted.

Remove the bowl and allow cooling for 1 minute only to warm the cheese but not cool completely. Mix in the egg yolk until well combined.

Lay parchment paper on a flat surface, pour the cheese mixture on top and cover with another parchment paper. Using a rolling pin, flatten the dough into 1/8-inch thickness.

Take off the parchment paper and cut the dough into spaghetti strands. Place in a bowl and refrigerate overnight.

When ready to cook, bring 2 cups of water to a boil in a medium saucepan and add the pasta. Cook for 40 seconds to 1 minute and then drain through a colander. Run cold water over the pasta and set aside to cool.

For the Mediterranean meatballs: (which can be made before cooking the pasta)

In a large pot, heat the olive oil and sauté the onions until softened, 3 minutes. Stir in the garlic and cook until fragrant, 30 seconds.

Stir in the tomato paste, tomatoes, saffron, and cinnamon sticks; cook for 2 minutes and then mix in the chicken broth, salt, and black pepper. Simmer for 20 to 25 minutes while you make the meatballs.

In a large bowl, mix the pork rinds, beef, egg, almond milk, garlic, salt, black pepper, coriander, nutmeg powder, paprika, ginger paste, cumin powder, cayenne pepper, turmeric powder, cloves powder, cilantro, parsley, 3 tablespoons of scallions, and almond flour. Form 1-inch meatballs from the mixture.

Heat olive oil in a skillet and fry the meatballs until brown on all sides, 10 minutes. Put meatballs into the sauce, coat well with the sauce and continue cooking for 10 minutes. Divide the pasta onto serving plates and spoon the meatballs with sauce on top. Garnish with the feta cheese, remaining scallions and serve warm.

Nutritional info per serving:

Calories 996; Fats 56.2g; Net Carbs 40.4g; Protein 60.1g

Thai Beef Shirataki Stir-Fry

Thai flavors are essential for your recipe collection because of the play of vegetables and flavors that you get.

Total Time: 35 minutes | **Serving**: 4

Ingredients

For the angel hair shirataki:

2 (8 oz) packs angel hair shirataki

For the teriyaki beef base:

2 tbsp olive oil, divided
1 ¼ lb flank steak, cut into bite-size pieces
Salt and black pepper to taste
1 white onion, thinly sliced
1 red bell pepper, deseeded and sliced
1 cup sliced shiitake mushrooms
4 garlic cloves, minced
1 ½ cups fresh Thai basil leaves
2 tbsp toasted sesame seeds
1 tbsp chopped peanuts
1 tbsp chopped fresh scallions

For the sauce:

3 tbsp coconut aminos
2 tbsp fish sauce
1 tbsp hot sauce

Directions

For the angel hair shirataki:

Boil 2 cups of water in a medium pot over medium heat.

Strain the shirataki pasta through a colander and rinse very well under hot running water.

Allow proper draining and pour the shirataki pasta into the boiling water. Cook for 3 minutes and strain again.

Place a dry skillet over medium heat and stir-fry the shirataki pasta until visibly dry, and makes a squeaky sound when stirred, 1 to 2 minutes. Take off the heat and set aside.

For the teriyaki beef base:

Heat the olive oil in a large skillet, season the meat with salt, black pepper, and sear in the oil on both sides until brown, 5 minutes. Transfer to a plate and set aside.

Add onion, bell pepper, and mushrooms to the skillet; cook for 5 minutes. Stir in the garlic and cook until fragrant, 1 minute. Return the beef to the skillet and add the pasta.

Quickly, combine the sauce's ingredients in a small bowl: coconut aminos, fish sauce, and hot sauce. Pour the mixture over the beef mix. Top with the Thai basil and toss well to coat. Cook for 1 to 2 minutes or until warmed through. Dish the food onto serving plates and garnish with the sesame seeds, peanuts, and scallions.

Nutritional info per serving:
Calories 358; Fats 16.8g; Net Carbs 15.8g; Protein 30.1g

Beef Ragu with Veggie Pasta

This time work some bell pepper noodles into your classic beef ragu and you will be testifying for long.

Total Time: 20 minutes | **Serving**: 4

Ingredients

2 tbsp butter
1 lb ground beef
Salt and black pepper to taste
1/4 cup sugar-free tomato sauce
4 tbsp chopped fresh parsley + extra for garnishing
4 green bell peppers, spiralized
4 red bell peppers, spiralized
1 small red onion, spiralized
1 cup grated Parmesan cheese

Directions

Heat half of the butter in a medium skillet and cook the beef until brown, 5 minutes. Season with salt and black pepper.

Stir in the tomato sauce, parsley, and cook for 10 minutes or until the sauce reduces by a quarter. Stir in the bell pepper and onion noodles; cook for 1 minute and turn the heat off.

Adjust the taste with salt, black pepper, and dish the food onto serving plates. Garnish with the Parmesan cheese and more parsley; serve warm.

Nutritional info per serving:
Calories 451; Fats 25.7g; Net Carbs 6.6g; Protein 39.8g

Classic Beef Lasagna

Anyone up for lasagna tonight? This classic is one to make!

Total Time: 70 minutes | **Serving**: 4

Ingredients

For the lasagna noodles:

4 oz cream cheese, room temperature
1 ½ cup grated mozzarella cheese

1 tsp dried Italian seasoning
2 large eggs, cracked into a bowl

For the lasagna filling:

1 lb ground beef
1 medium white onion, chopped
1 tsp Italian seasoning
Salt and black pepper to taste

1 cup sugar-free marinara sauce
6 tbsp ricotta cheese
½ cup grated mozzarella cheese
½ cup grated Parmesan cheese

Directions

For the lasagna noodles:

Preheat the oven to 350 F and line a 9 x 13 –inch baking sheet with parchment paper.

In a food processor, add cream cheese, mozzarella cheese, Italian seasoning, and eggs. Blend until well mixed. Pour the cheese mixture on the baking sheet and spread across the pan. Bake until set and firm to touch, 20 minutes. Remove and let cool.

For the lasagna sauce:

In a large skillet, combine the beef, onion and cook until brown, 5 minutes. Season with the Italian seasoning, salt, and black pepper. Cook further for 1 minute and mix in the marinara sauce. Simmer for 3 minutes. Turn the heat off.

Evenly cut the lasagna pasta into thirds making sure it fits into your baking sheet. Spread a layer of the beef mixture in the baking sheet and make a first single layer on the beef mixture. Spread a third of the remaining beef mixture on the pasta, top with a third each of the ricotta cheese, mozzarella cheese, and Parmesan cheese. Repeat the layering two more times using the remaining ingredients in the same quantities.

Bake in the oven until the cheese melts and is bubbly with the sauce, 20 minutes. Remove the lasagna, allow cooling for 2 minutes and dish onto serving plates. Serve warm.

Nutritional info per serving:

Calories 557; Fats 29.6g; Net Carbs 4.6g; Protein 60.2g

Creamy Sun-Dried & Parsnip Noodles

This dish reminds of Italian foods. If we are talking about pasta, then this one is deserving of its place.

Total Time: 35 minutes | **Serving**: 4

Ingredients

3 tbsp butter
1 lb beef stew meat, cut into strips
Salt and black pepper to taste
4 large parsnips, spiralized
1 cup sun dried tomatoes in oil, chopped
4 garlic cloves, minced
1 ¼ cup heavy cream
1 cup shaved Parmesan cheese
¼ tsp dried basil
¼ tsp red chili flakes
2 tbsp chopped fresh parsley for garnishing

Directions

Melt 1 tablespoon of butter in a large skillet, season the beef with salt, black pepper and cook in the butter until brown, and cooked within, 8 to 10 minutes.

In another medium skillet, melt the remaining butter and sauté the parsnips until softened, 5 to 7 minutes. Set aside.

Stir in the sun-dried tomatoes and garlic into the beef, cook until fragrant, 1 minute.

Reduce the heat to low and stir in the heavy cream and Parmesan cheese. Simmer until the cheese melts. Season with the salt, basil, and red chili flakes.

Fold in the parsnips until well coated and cook for 2 more minutes.

Dish the food into serving plates, garnish with the parsley and serve warm.

Nutritional info per serving:

Calories 596; Fats 34.8g; Net Carbs 16.7g; Protein 36.8g

Keto Beef Carbonara

Pasta and carbonara are a heavenly match and should be enjoyed often on the keto diet.

Total Time: 30 minutes + chilling time | **Serving**: 4

Ingredients

For the keto pasta:

1 cup shredded mozzarella cheese

1 large egg yolk

For the carbonara:

4 bacon slices, chopped

1¼ cups heavy whipping cream

¼ cup mayonnaise

Salt and black pepper to taste

4 egg yolks

1 cup grated Parmesan cheese

Directions

For the pasta:

Pour cheese into a safe-microwave bowl and melt in the microwave for 2 minutes while stirring at 20-second intervals until fully melted. Allow cooling for 1 minute only to warm the cheese but not cool completely. Mix in the egg yolk until well combined.

Lay a parchment paper on a flat surface, pour the cheese mixture on top and cover with another parchment paper. Using a rolling pin, flatten the dough into 1/8-inch thickness. Take off the parchment paper and cut the dough into thin spaghetti strands. Place in a bowl and refrigerate overnight. Bring 2 cups of water to a boil in a saucepan and add pasta. Cook for 1 minute and then drain. Run cold water over and set aside to cool.

For the carbonara:

Add the bacon to a skillet and cook over medium heat until crispy, 5 minutes. Set aside. Pour heavy cream into a pot and allow simmering for 5 minutes. Whisk in mayonnaise and season with the salt and pepper. Cook for 1 minute and spoon 2 tablespoons of the mixture into a medium bowl. Allow cooling and mix in the egg yolks.

Pour the mixture into the pot and mix quickly until well combined. Stir in Parmesan cheese and fold in the pasta. Garnish with more Parmesan cheese. Cook for 1 minute to warm the pasta.

Nutritional info per serving:

Calories 470; Fats 35.5g; Net Carbs 8.9g; Protein 25.4g

PORK

Pesto Parmesan Pork with Green Pasta

Basil, pine nuts and lots of olive oil is excellent for any pasta dish. I love this combo!

Total Time: 1 hour 27 minutes | **Serving**: 4

Ingredients
4 boneless pork chops
Salt and black pepper to taste
½ cup basil pesto, olive oil-based
1 cup grated Parmesan cheese
1 tbsp butter
4 large turnips, spiralized

Directions
Preheat the oven to 350 F.

Season the pork with salt, black pepper and place on a baking sheet. Divide the pesto on top and spread well on the pork.

Place the sheet in the oven and bake for 45 minutes to 1 hour or until cooked through.

When ready, pull out the baking sheet and divide half of the Parmesan cheese on top of the pork. Cook further for 10 minutes or until the cheese melts. Remove the pork and set aside for serving.

Melt the butter in a medium skillet and sauté the turnips until tender, 5 to 7 minutes. Stir in the remaining Parmesan cheese and divide between serving plates.

Top with the pork and serve warm.

Nutritional info per serving:
Calories 532; Fats 28.4g; Net Carbs 4.9g; Protein 53.8g

Pork Lo Mein

Are you up for more Asian flavors? This pasta-veggie mix is one to have frequently.

Total Time: 25 minutes + overtime chilling time | **Serving**: 4

Ingredients

For the keto pasta:

1 cup shredded mozzarella cheese
1 egg yolk

For the pork and vegetables:

1 tbsp sesame oil
3 boneless pork chops, cut into ¼-inch strips
Salt and black pepper to taste
1 red bell pepper, deseeded and thinly sliced
1 yellow bell pepper, deseeded and thinly sliced
1 cup green beans, trimmed and halved
1 garlic clove, minced
1-inch ginger knob, peeled and grated
4 green onions, chopped
1 tsp toasted sesame seeds to garnish

For the sauce:

3 tbsp coconut aminos
2 tsp sesame oil
2 tsp sugar-free maple syrup
1 tsp fresh ginger paste

Directions

For the pasta:

Pour the cheese into a medium safe-microwave bowl and melt in the microwave for 2 minutes while stirring at 20-second intervals until fully melted.

Take out the bowl and allow cooling for 1 minute only to warm the cheese but not cool completely. Mix in the egg yolk until well-combined.

Lay a parchment paper on a flat surface, pour the cheese mixture on top and cover with another parchment paper. Using a rolling pin, flatten the dough into 1/8-inch thickness. Take off the parchment paper and cut the dough into thin spaghetti strands. Place in a bowl and refrigerate overnight.

When ready to cook, bring 2 cups of water to a boil in medium saucepan and add the pasta. Cook for 40 seconds to 1 minute and then drain through a colander. Run cold water over the pasta and set aside to cool.

For the pork and vegetables:

Heat the sesame oil in a large skillet, season the pork with salt, black pepper, and sear in the oil on both sides until brown, 5 minutes. Transfer to a plate and set aside.

Mix in the bell peppers, green beans and cook until sweaty, 3 minutes. Stir in the garlic, ginger, green onions and cook until fragrant, 1 minute.

Add the pork and pasta to the skillet and toss well.

In a small bowl, toss the sauce's ingredients the coconut aminos, sesame oil, maple syrup, and ginger paste.

Pour the mixture over the pork mixture and toss well; cook for 1 minute.

Dish the food onto serving plates and garnish with the sesame seeds. Serve warm.

Nutritional info per serving:

Calories 338; Fats 12.6g; Net Carbs 4.6g; Protein 43g

Pasta & Cheese Pulled Pork

Now, this looks more like a regular mac and cheese but tastier and healthier than the traditional type.

Total Time: 1 hour 45 minutes + overtime chilling time | **Serving**: 4

Ingredients

For the keto macaroni:

1 cup shredded mozzarella cheese
1 egg yolk

For the pulled pork mac and cheese:

2 tbsp olive oil
1 lb pork shoulders, divided into 3 pieces
Salt and black pepper to taste
1 tsp dried thyme
1 cup chicken broth
2 tbsp butter
2 medium shallots, minced
2 garlic cloves, minced
1 cup water
1 cup grated Monterey Jack cheese
4 oz cream cheese, room temperature
1 cup heavy cream
½ tsp white pepper
½ tsp nutmeg powder
2 tbsp chopped parsley

Directions

For the keto macaroni:

Pour the cheese into a medium safe-microwave bowl and melt in the microwave for 2 minutes while stirring at 20-second intervals until fully melted.

Take out the bowl and allow cooling for 1 minute only to warm the cheese but not cool completely. Mix in the egg yolk until well-combined.

Lay a parchment paper on a flat surface, pour the cheese mixture on top and cover with another parchment paper. Using a rolling pin, flatten the dough into 1/8-inch thickness.

Take off the parchment paper and cut the dough into small cubes of the size of macaroni. Place in a bowl and refrigerate overnight.

When ready to cook, bring 2 cups of water to a boil in medium saucepan and add the keto macaroni. Cook for 40 seconds to 1 minute and then drain through a colander. Run cold water over the pasta and set aside to cool.

For the pulled pork mac and cheese:

Heat the olive oil in a large pot, season the pork with salt, black pepper, thyme, and sear in the oil on both sides until brown. Pour on the chicken broth, cover, and cook over low heat for 45 minutes to 1 hour or until softened. When ready, remove the pork onto a plate and shred into small strands. Set aside.

Preheat the oven to 380 F.

Melt the butter in a large skillet and sauté the shallots until softened. Stir in the garlic and cook until fragrant, 30 seconds.

Pour in the water to deglaze the pot and then stir in half of the Monterey Jack cheese and cream cheese until melted, 4 minutes. Mix in the heavy cream and season with salt, black pepper, white pepper, and nutmeg powder.

Add the pasta, pork, and half of the parsley to the mixture; combine well.

Pour the mixture into a baking dish and cover the top with the remaining Monterey Jack cheese. Bake in the oven until the cheese melts and the food bubbly, 15 to 20 minutes.

Remove from the oven, allow cooling for 2 minutes and garnish with the parsley.

Serve warm.

Nutritional info per serving:

Calories 603; Fats 43.6g; Net Carbs 1.5g; Protein 45.9g

Creamy Pork with Green Beans and Keto Fettuccine

I love the crunch that green beans give this creamy pork dish. Something unique for a difference!

Total Time: 40 minutes + overtime chilling time | **Serving**: 4

Ingredients

For the keto fettuccine:

1 cup shredded mozzarella cheese

1 egg yolk

For the creamy pork and green beans:

1 tbsp olive oil

4 pork loin medallions, cut into thin strips

Salt and black pepper to taste

½ cup green beans, chopped

1 lemon, zested and juiced

¼ cup chicken broth

1 cup crème fraiche

6 basil leaves, chopped

1 cup shaved Parmesan cheese for topping

Directions

For the keto fettucine:

Pour the cheese into a medium safe-microwave bowl and melt in the microwave for 2 minutes while stirring at 20-second intervals until fully melted. Take out the bowl and allow cooling for 1 minute only to warm the cheese but not cool completely. Mix in the egg yolk until well-combined.

Lay a parchment paper on a flat surface, pour the cheese mixture on top and cover with another parchment paper. Using a rolling pin, flatten the dough into 1/8-inch thickness. Take off the parchment paper and cut the dough into thick fettuccine strands. Place in a bowl and refrigerate overnight. Bring 2 cups of water to a boil in a saucepan and add keto fettuccine. Cook for 1 minute and then drain. Set aside to cool.

For the creamy pork and green beans:

Heat olive oil in a skillet, season the pork with salt, pepper, and cook for 10 minutes. Mix in green beans and cook for 5 minutes. Stir in lemon zest, lemon juice, and chicken broth. Cook for 5 more minutes or until the liquid reduces by a quarter. Add crème fraiche and mix well. Pour in pasta and basil and cook for 1 minute. Top with Parmesan.

Nutritional info per serving:

Calories 586; Fats 32.3g; Net Carbs 9g; Protein 59g

Delicious Sambal Pork Noodles

Sambal noodles may not be common to you but the aroma and taste will make you have it more often.

Total Time: 60 minutes | **Serving**: 4

Ingredients

For the shirataki noodles:

2 (8 oz) packs Miracle noodles, garlic and herb
Salt to season

For the sambal pork:

1 tbsp olive oil
1 lb ground pork
4 garlic cloves, minced
1-inch ginger, peeled and grated
1 tsp liquid stevia
1 tbsp sugar-free tomato paste
2 fresh basil leaves + extra for garnishing
2 tbsp sambal oelek
2 tbsp plain vinegar
1 cup water
2 tbsp coconut aminos
Salt to taste
1 tbsp unsalted butter

Directions

For the shirataki noodles:

Bring 2 cups of water to a boil in a pot over medium heat. Strain the Miracle noodles and rinse very well under hot running water. Allow proper draining and pour the noodles into the boiling water. Take off the heat and let sit for 3 minutes and strain again.

Place a dry skillet over medium heat and stir-fry the shirataki noodles until visibly dry, 1 to 2 minutes. Season with salt, plate and set aside.

For the pork sambal:

Heat the olive oil in a large pot and cook in the pork until brown, 5 minutes. Stir in the garlic, ginger, liquid stevia and cook for 1 minute. Add in tomato paste, cook for 2 minutes and mix in basil, sambal oelek, vinegar, water, coconut aminos, and salt. Cover the pot and continue cooking for 30 minutes. Uncover, add the shirataki noodles, butter and mix well into the sauce. Garnish with some basil leaves and serve warm.

Nutritional info per serving:

Calories 505; Fats 30.2g; Net Carbs 22.1g; Protein 33.9g

Lemongrass Pork with Spaghetti Squash

Lemongrass gives this dish a special hint and who knew that it will pair well with spaghetti squash?

Total Time: 1 hour + marinating time | **Serving**: 4

Ingredients

For the lemongrass pork:

2 tbsp minced lemongrass
2 tbsp fresh ginger paste
2 tbsp sugar-free maple syrup
2 tbsp coconut aminos
1 tbsp fish sauce
4 boneless pork chops
2 tbsp peanut oil

For the squash noodles:

3 lb spaghetti squashes, halved and deseeded
1 tbsp olive oil
Salt and black pepper to taste

For the steamed spinach:

1 tbsp peanut oil
1 tsp fresh ginger paste
1 lb baby spinach

For the peanut-coconut sauce:

½ cup coconut milk
¼ cup organic peanut butter

Directions

For the lemongrass pork:

In a medium bowl, mix the lemongrass, ginger paste, maple syrup, coconut aminos, and fish sauce. Place the pork in the liquid and coat well. Allow marinating for 45 minutes.

After, heat the peanut oil in a large skillet, remove the pork from the marinade and sear in the oil on both sides until golden brown and cooked through, 10 to 15 minutes. Transfer to a plate and cover with foil.

For the spaghetti squash:

Preheat the oven to 380 F.

Place the spaghetti squashes on a baking sheet, brush with the olive oil and season with salt and black pepper. Bake in the oven for 20 to 25 minutes or until tender.

When ready, remove the squash and shred with two forks into spaghetti-like strands. Keep warm in the oven.

For the spinach:

In another skillet, heat the peanut oil and sauté the ginger until fragrant. Add the spinach and cook to wilt while stirring to be coated well in the ginger, 2 minutes.

For the peanut-coconut sauce:

In a medium bowl, quickly whisk the coconut milk with the peanut butter until well combined.

To serve:

Unwrap and divide the pork into four bowls, add the spaghetti squash to the side, then the spinach and drizzle the peanut sauce on top.

Serve immediately.

Nutritional info per serving:
Calories 694; Fats 34.1g; Net Carbs 37.1g; Protein 53.6g

Pork Avocado Keto Noodles

A classic that works excellently for the entire family whether on the keto diet or not.

Total Time: 15 minutes | **Serving**: 4

Ingredients

2 tbsp butter
1 lb ground pork
Salt and black pepper to taste
8 red and yellow bell peppers, spiralized
1 tsp garlic powder
2 medium avocados, pitted, peeled and mashed
2 tbsp chopped pecans for topping

Directions

Melt the butter in a large skillet and cook the pork until brown, 5 minutes. Season with salt and black pepper. Stir in the bell peppers, garlic powder and cook until the peppers are slightly tender, 2 minutes.

Mix in the mashed avocados, adjust the taste with salt and black pepper and cook for 1 minute. Dish the food onto serving plates, garnish with the pecans and serve warm.

Nutritional info per serving:
Calories 704; Fats 49.5g; Net Carbs 22.3g; Protein 35.8g

Chinese Pork and Celeriac Noodles

One of my favorite cuisines is the Chinese one and this dish is one of my favorites.

Total Time: 1 hour 18 minutes | **Serving**: 4

Ingredients

3 tbsp sugar-free maple syrup
3 tbsp coconut aminos
1 tbsp fresh ginger paste
¼ tsp Chinese five spice powder
Salt and black pepper to taste
1 lb pork tenderloin, cut into 1-inch cubes
2 tbsp butter
4 medium large celeriac, spiralized
1 tbsp sesame oil
4 heads baby bok choy, leaves separated
2 green onions, chopped for garnishing
2 tbsp sesame seeds for garnishing

Directions

Preheat the oven to 400 F and line a baking sheet with foil.

In a large bowl, mix the maple syrup, coconut aminos, ginger paste, Chinese five-spice powder, salt, and black pepper. Spoon 3 tablespoons of the mixture into a small bowl and reserve for topping. Mix the pork cubes into the remaining marinade and set aside to marinate for 25 minutes.

Meanwhile, melt the butter in a medium skillet and sauté the celeriac until softened, 5 to 7 minutes or until tender. Turn the heat off and set aside.

When the marinating is over, remove the pork from the marinade onto the baking sheet and cook in the oven for 40 minutes or until cooked through.

When the pork is almost ready, heat the sesame oil in a large skillet and sauté the bok choy and zucchini pasta until slightly wilted and tender, 2 to 3 minutes.

Transfer to serving bowls and top with the pork when ready. Garnish with the green onions and sesame seeds. Drizzle the reserved marinade on top and serve warm.

Nutritional info per serving:

Calories 409; Fats 17.8g; Net Carbs 3g; Protein 44.5g

Garlic Pecorino Kohlrabi with Sausage

Incorporate some pork sausages into your zoodles, which makes it kid-friendly for full family servings.

Total Time: 15 minutes | **Serving**: 4

Ingredients

2 tbsp olive oil
1 cup sliced pork sausage
4 bacon slices, chopped
4 large kohlrabi, spiralized
6 garlic cloves, minced
1 cup cherry tomatoes, halved
Salt and black pepper to taste
7 fresh basil leaves
1 cup grated Pecorino Romano cheese
1 tbsp pine nuts for topping

Directions

Heat the olive oil in a large skillet and cook the sausage and bacon until brown, 5 minutes. Transfer to a plate and set aside.

Stir in the kohlrabi and cook until tender, 5 to 7 minutes. Mix the garlic into the oil and cook until fragrant, 30 seconds. Then, add the cherry tomatoes, salt, and black pepper; cook for 2 minutes.

Mix in the sausage, bacon, basil, and half of the Pecorino Romano cheese. Turn the heat off.

Dish the food onto serving plates and garnish with the remaining cheese and pine nuts.

Serve warm.

Nutritional info per serving:

Calories 229; Fats 20.2g; Net Carbs 2.43g; Protein 7.6g

CHICKEN

Chicken Alfredo Zoodles

Do you prefer chicken for your alfredo? This one with zoodles is highly recommended.

Total Time: 23 minutes | **Serving**: 4

Ingredients
4 tbsp butter
4 boneless chicken breasts, cut into 1-inch cubes
Salt and black pepper to taste
4 large turnips, spiralized
3 garlic cloves, minced
¾ cup heavy cream
1 cup grated Pecorino Romano cheese
2 tbsp chopped fresh parsley

Directions
Melt 2 tablespoons of butter in a large skillet, season the chicken with salt, black pepper, and cook in the oil until golden brown on both sides and cooked within, 10 minutes. Transfer to a plate and set aside.

Melt the remaining butter in the skillet and sauté the turnips until softened, 6 minutes.

Add the garlic to the pan and cook until fragrant, 1 minute.

Reduce the heat to low and stir in the heavy cream and Pecorino Romano cheese until melted. Season with salt, black pepper.

Stir in the chicken and dish the food onto serving plates.

Garnish with the parsley and serve warm.

Nutritional info per serving:
Calories 771; Fats 49.2g; Net Carbs 2.3g; Protein 68.6g

One-Pot Spicy Cheddar Pasta

One that I would recommend for lunch – enough chili to boost your mood.

Total Time: 35 minutes | **Serving**: 4

Ingredients

For the shirataki fettuccine:

2 (8 oz) packs shirataki fettuccine

For the spicy cheddar pasta:

4 chicken breasts
1 medium yellow onion, minced
3 garlic cloves, minced
1 tsp Italian seasoning
½ tsp garlic powder
¼ tsp red chili flakes
¼ tsp cayenne pepper
1 cup sugar-free marinara sauce
1 cup grated mozzarella cheese
½ cup grated cheddar cheese
Salt and black pepper to taste
2 tbsp chopped parsley

Directions

For the shirataki fettuccine:

Boil 2 cups of water in a medium pot over medium heat. Strain the shirataki pasta and rinse very well under hot running water. Allow proper draining and pour the shirataki pasta into the boiling water. Take off the heat and let sit for 3 minutes and strain again.

Place a dry skillet over medium heat and stir-fry the shirataki pasta until visibly dry, and makes a squeaky sound when stirred, 1 to 2 minutes. Take off the heat and set aside.

For the spicy cheddar pasta:

Heat the olive oil in a large pot, season the chicken with salt, black pepper, and cook in the oil until golden brown on both sides and cooked within, 10 minutes. Transfer to a plate, cut into cubes and set aside. Add the onion and garlic to the pan and cook until softened and fragrant, 3 minutes. Season with the Italian seasoning, garlic powder, red chili flakes, and cayenne pepper. Cook for 1 minute.

Stir in marinara sauce and simmer for 5 minutes. Adjust the taste with salt and black pepper. Reduce heat to low and return the chicken to the sauce and shirataki fettucine, mozzarella and cheddar cheeses. Stir until the cheese melts. Garnish with parsley.

Nutritional info per serving:

Calories 763; Fats 34g; Net Carbs 17.9g; Protein 82.7g

Creamy Tuscan Chicken Linguine

I love incorporating classics whenever I can and this Italian one serves well.

Total Time: 35 minutes + overtime chilling time | **Serving**: 4

Ingredients

For the keto linguine:

1 cup shredded mozzarella cheese
1 egg yolk

For the creamy Tuscan chicken:

2 tbsp olive oil
4 chicken breasts
1 medium white onion, chopped
1 cup sundried tomatoes in oil, drained and chopped
1 red bell pepper, deseeded and chopped
5 garlic cloves, minced
1 tsp dried oregano
¾ cup chicken broth
1 ½ cup heavy cream
¾ cup grated Pecorino Romano cheese
1 cup baby kale, chopped
Salt and black pepper to taste

Directions

For the keto linguine:

Pour the cheese into a medium safe-microwave bowl and melt in the microwave for 2 minutes while stirring at 20-second intervals until fully melted. Take out the bowl and allow cooling for 1 minute only to warm the cheese but not cool completely. Mix in the egg yolk until well-combined.

Lay a parchment paper on a flat surface, pour the cheese mixture on top and cover with another parchment paper. Using a rolling pin, flatten the dough into 1/8-inch thickness.

Take off the parchment paper and cut the dough into linguine-like strands. Place in a bowl and refrigerate overnight.

When ready to cook, bring 2 cups of water to a boil in medium saucepan and add the keto linguine. Cook for 40 seconds to 1 minute and then drain through a colander. Run cold water over the pasta and set aside to cool.

For the creamy Tuscan chicken:

Heat the olive oil in a large skillet, season the chicken with salt, black pepper, and cook in the oil until golden brown on the outside and cooked within, 7 to 8 minutes. Transfer the chicken to a plate and cut into 4 slices each. Set aside.

Add the onion, sundried tomatoes, bell pepper to the skillet and sauté until softened, 5 minutes. Mix in the garlic, oregano and cook until fragrant, 1 minute.

Deglaze the skillet with the chicken broth and mix in the heavy cream. Simmer for 2 minutes and stir in the Pecorino Romano cheese until melted, 2 minutes.

Once the cheese melts, stir in the kale to wilt and adjust the taste with salt and black pepper.

Mix in the linguine and chicken until well coated in the sauce.

Dish the food and serve warm.

Nutritional info per serving:
Calories 941; Fats 60.7g; Net Carbs 10.7g; Protein 79.3g

Tomato Kale Chicken Skillet with Keto Linguine

While this would have been a regular vegetable sauce with keto pasta, adding Parmesan cheese makes it keto-certified and yummier.

Total Time: 30 minutes + overnight chilling time | **Serving**: 4

Ingredients

For the keto linguine:

1 cup shredded mozzarella cheese

1 egg yolk

For the tomato-kale chicken:

3 tbsp olive oil
4 chicken thighs, cut into 1-inch pieces
Salt and black pepper to taste
1 yellow onion, chopped
4 garlic cloves, minced
1 cup cherry tomatoes, halved
½ cup chicken broth
2 cups baby kale, chopped
1 cup grated Parmigiano-Reggiano cheese for serving
2 tbsp pine nuts for topping

Directions

For the keto linguine:

Pour the cheese into a medium safe-microwave bowl and melt in the microwave for 2 minutes while stirring at 20-second intervals until fully melted.

Take out the bowl and allow cooling for 1 minute only to warm the cheese but not cool completely. Mix in the egg yolk until well-combined.

Lay a parchment paper on a flat surface, pour the cheese mixture on top and cover with another parchment paper. Using a rolling pin, flatten the dough into 1/8-inch thickness.

Take off the parchment paper and cut the dough into linguine strands. Place in a bowl and refrigerate overnight.

When ready to cook, bring 2 cups of water to a boil in medium saucepan and add the keto linguine. Cook for 40 seconds to 1 minute and then drain through a colander. Run cold water over the pasta and set aside to cool.

For the tomato-kale chicken:

Heat the olive oil in a medium pot, season the chicken with salt, black pepper, and sear in the oil until golden brown on the outside. Transfer to a plate and set aside.

Add the onion and garlic to the oil and cook until softened and fragrant, 3 minutes.

Mix in the tomatoes and chicken broth, cover and cook over low heat until the tomatoes soften and the liquid reduces by half. Season with salt and black pepper.

Return the chicken to the pot and stir in the kale. Allow wilting for 2 minutes.

Divide the keto linguine onto serving plates, top with the kale sauce and then the Parmigianino-Reggiano cheese.

Garnish with the pine nuts and serve warm.

Nutritional info per serving:

Calories 740; Fats 52.9g; Carbs 15.1g; Net Carbs 6.1g; Protein 50.2g

Cajun Chicken Fettuccine

Traditional American flavors anyone? Here's one for you to splurge!

Total Time: 45 minutes + overnight chilling time| **Serving**: 4

Ingredients

For the keto fettuccine:

1 cup shredded mozzarella cheese
1 egg yolk

For the Cajun chicken:

2 tbsp olive oil
4 chicken breasts, cut into 1-inch cubes
1 medium yellow onion, thinly sliced
1 medium red bell pepper, deseeded and thinly sliced
1 medium green bell pepper, deseeded and thinly sliced
4 garlic cloves, minced
4 tsp Cajun seasoning
1 cup sugar-free Alfredo sauce
½ cup sugar-free marinara sauce
2 cups grated mozzarella cheese
½ cup grated Parmesan cheese
2 tbsp chopped fresh parsley

Directions

For the keto fettucine:

Pour the cheese into a medium safe-microwave bowl and melt in the microwave for 2 minutes while stirring at 20-second intervals until fully melted.

Take out the bowl and allow cooling for 1 minute only to warm the cheese but not cool completely. Mix in the egg yolk until well-combined.

Lay a parchment paper on a flat surface, pour the cheese mixture on top and cover with another parchment paper. Using a rolling pin, flatten the dough into 1/8-inch thickness.

Take off the parchment paper and cut the dough into thick fettuccine strands. Place in a bowl and refrigerate overnight. When ready to cook, bring 2 cups of water to a boil in medium saucepan and add the keto fettuccine. Cook for 40 seconds to 1 minute and then drain through a colander. Run cold water over the pasta and set aside to cool.

For the Cajun chicken:

Preheat the oven to 350 F and grease a baking dish with cooking spray.

Heat the olive oil in a medium skillet, season the chicken with salt, and black pepper, cook in the oil until seared on the outside, 6 minutes. Transfer to a plate.

Add the onion and bell peppers to the skillet and cook until softened, 5 minutes. Stir in the garlic and cook until fragrant, 30 seconds.

Return the chicken to the pot and stir in the Cajun seasoning, Alfredo sauce, and marinara sauce. Cook for 3 minutes over low heat.

Stir in the keto fettuccine until well-coated in the sauce and transfer the mixture to the baking dish.

Cover with the mozzarella and Parmesan cheeses, and bake in the oven until the cheeses melt and are golden brown on top, 15 minutes.

Remove from the oven, garnish with the parsley and serve warm.

Nutritional info per serving:

Calories 777; Fats 38.3g; Net Carbs 4.6g; Protein 92.8g

Saffron Chicken and Pasta

Are you torn between an Indian and Mediterranean blend? This dish will bring some difference to your culinary lifestyle.

Total Time: 35 minutes + overnight chilling time| **Serving**: 4

Ingredients

For the keto fettuccine:

1 cup shredded mozzarella cheese
1 egg yolk

For the saffron chicken:

3 tbsp butter
4 chicken breasts, cut into strips
½ tsp ground saffron threads
1 yellow onion, finely chopped
2 garlic cloves, minced
1 tbsp almond flour
1 pinch cardamom powder
1 pinch cinnamon powder
1 cup heavy cream
1 cup chicken stock
¼ cup chopped scallions
3 tbsp chopped parsley
Salt and black pepper to taste

Directions

For the keto fettuccine:

Pour the cheese into a medium safe-microwave bowl and melt in the microwave for 2 minutes while stirring at 20-second intervals until fully melted.

Take out the bowl and allow cooling for 1 minute only to warm the cheese but not cool completely. Mix in the egg yolk until well-combined.

Lay a parchment paper on a flat surface, pour the cheese mixture on top and cover with another parchment paper. Using a rolling pin, flatten the dough into 1/8-inch thickness.

Take off the parchment paper and cut the dough into thick fettuccine strands. Place in a bowl and refrigerate overnight.

When ready to cook, bring 2 cups of water to a boil in medium saucepan and add the keto fettuccine. Cook for 40 seconds to 1 minute and then drain through a colander. Run cold water over the pasta and set aside to cool.

For the saffron chicken:

Melt the butter in a large skillet, season the chicken with salt, black pepper, and cook in the oil until golden brown on the outside, 5 minutes.

Stir in the saffron, onion, garlic and cook until the onion softens and the garlic and saffron are fragrant, 3 minutes.

Stir in the almond flour, cardamom powder, cinnamon powder, and cook for 1 minute to exude some fragrance.

Add the heavy cream, chicken stock and cook for 2 to 3 minutes.

Adjust the taste with salt, black pepper and mix in the keto fettucine and scallions. Allow warming for 1 to 2 minutes and turn the heat off.

Dish the food onto serving plates and garnish with the parsley.

Serve warm.

Nutritional info per serving:

Calories 775; Fats 48.1g; Net Carbs 3.1g; Protein 73.4g

Mustard Chicken Shirataki

The sharp flavor of mustard is evident in this mix. I love it! You may swap wholegrain mustard with Dijon mustard if you want a switch in flavor-intensity.

Total Time: 40 minutes | **Serving**: 4

Ingredients

For the shirataki angel hair:

2 (8 oz) packs angel hair shirataki

For the mustard chicken sauce:

- 1 tbsp olive oil
- 4 chicken breasts, cut into strips
- Salt and black pepper to taste
- 1 yellow onion, finely sliced
- 1 yellow bell pepper, deseeded and sliced
- 1 garlic clove, minced
- 1 tbsp wholegrain mustard
- 5 tbsp heavy cream
- 1 cup chopped mustard greens
- 1 tbsp chopped parsley

Directions

For the shirataki angel hair:

Boil 2 cups of water in a medium pot over medium heat. Srain the shirataki pasta and rinse very well under hot running water. Allow proper draining and pour the shirataki pasta into the boiling water. Take off the heat and let sit for 3 minutes and strain again. Place a dry skillet over medium heat and stir-fry the shirataki pasta until visibly dry, and makes a squeaky sound when stirred, 1 to 2 minutes. Take off the heat and set aside.

For the mustard chicken sauce:

Heat the olive oil in a large skillet, season the chicken with salt, black pepper, and cook in the oil until golden brown, 10 minutes. Set aside. Stir in the onion, bell pepper and cook until softened, 5 minutes. Mix in the garlic and cook until fragrant, 30 seconds.

Mix in the mustard and heavy cream; simmer for 2 minutes and mix in the chicken and mustard greens. Allow wilting for 2 minutes and adjust the taste with salt and black pepper.

Stir in the shirataki pasta, allow warming for 1 minute and dish the food onto serving plates. Garnish with the parsley and serve warm.

Nutritional info per serving:

Calories 692; Fats 38.3g; Net Carbs 15.7g; Protein 64.8g

VEGETABLES

Creamy Mushrooms with Broccoli Pasta

Mushrooms replace meat dishes excellently and there was no better way to kick off this section than with mushrooms.

Total Time: 20 minutes | **Serving**: 4

Ingredients
4 large broccoli
2 tbsp olive oil
1 cup sliced cremini mushrooms
2 garlic cloves, minced
4 scallions, chopped
2 tbsp almond flour
1 ½ cups almond milk
2/3 cup grated Gruyere cheese
Salt and black pepper to taste
¼ cup chopped fresh parsley

Directions

Cut off the florets of the broccoli heads leaving only the stems. Cut the ends of the stem flatly and evenly. Run the stems through a spiralizer to make the noodles.

Heat the olive oil in a large skillet and sauté the broccoli noodles and mushrooms until softened, 5 to 7 minutes. Stir in the garlic and scallions; cook until fragrant, 1 minute.

In a medium bowl, combine the almond flour and almond milk, and pour the mixture over the vegetables. Stir and allow thickening for 2 to 3 minutes.

Whisk in half of the Gruyere cheese to melt and adjust the taste with salt and black pepper.

Dish the food onto serving plates, garnish with the remaining Gruyere cheese and parsley. Serve warm.

Nutritional info per serving:
Calories 221; Fats 15.6g; Net Carbs 1.41g; Protein 9.3g

Cauliflower Casserole with Shirataki

My kids love pasta bakes and I find that this cauliflower option works well for the entire family.

Total Time: 45 minutes | **Serving**: 4

Ingredients

For the shirataki angel hair:

2 (8 oz) packs spinach angel hair shirataki

For the casserole:

1 medium head cauliflower, cut into florets
1 cup heavy cream
1 cup grated Monterey Jack cheese
1 tsp dried thyme
1 tsp smoked paprika
Salt to taste
½ tsp red chili flakes

Directions

For the shirataki angel hair:

Boil 2 cups of water in a medium pot over medium heat. Strain the shirataki pasta through a colander and rinse very well under hot running water. Allow proper draining and pour the shirataki pasta into the boiling water. Take off the heat and let sit for 3 minutes and strain again.

Place a dry skillet over medium heat and stir-fry the shirataki pasta until visibly dry, and makes a squeaky sound when stirred, 1 to 2 minutes. Take off the heat and set aside.

For the casserole:

Preheat the oven to 350 F and grease a baking dish with cooking spray. Set aside.

Bring 4 cups of water to a boil in a large pot and blanch the cauliflower for 4 minutes. Drain through a colander.

In a large bowl, mix the cauliflower, shirataki, heavy cream, half of the Monterey Jack cheese, thyme, paprika, salt, and red chili flakes until well-combined.

Transfer the mixture to the baking dish and top with the remaining cheese.

Bake for 30 minutes. Allow cooling for 2 minutes and serve afterwards.

Nutritional info per serving:

Calories 301; Fats 20.8g; Net Carbs 13.4g; Protein 11.6g

Tofu Spaghetti Bolognese

A classic that won't only serve your dietary needs but one that the children will enjoy too

Total Time: 25 minutes | **Serving**: 4

Ingredients

For the pasta:

2 tbsp butter
4 large parsnips, spiralized
Salt to taste

For the tofu Bolognese:

2 tbsp olive oil
1 cup pressed and crumbled firm tofu
1 medium white onion, chopped
2 celery stalks, finely chopped
1 garlic clove, minced
1 bay leaf
2 cups sugar-free passata
¼ cup vegetable broth
Salt and black pepper to taste
1 small bunch basil, chopped
1 cup grated Parmesan cheese for topping

Directions

For the pasta:

Melt the butter in a medium skillet and sauté the parsnips until tender, 5 to 7 minutes. Season with salt and set aside for serving.

For the tofu Bolognese:

Heat the olive oil in a large pot and cook the tofu until brown, 5 minutes.

Stir in the onion, celery, and cook until softened, 5 minutes. Add the garlic, bay leaf and cook until fragrant, 30 seconds.

Mix in the passata, vegetable broth and season with salt and black pepper. Cover the pot and cook until the sauce thickens, 8 to 10 minutes.

Open the lid, stir in the basil and adjust the taste with salt and black pepper.

Divide the pasta onto serving plates and top with the Bolognese.

Sprinkle the Parmesan cheese on top and serve warm.

Nutritional info per serving:

Calories 424; Fats 19.8g; Net Carbs 30.9g; Protein 21.7g

Balsamic Veggie-Pasta Mix

Rather tangy for a keto diet but watch out for the cheese and nut topping at the end. It makes the difference!

Total Time: 25 minutes + overnight chilling time| **Serving**: 4

Ingredients

For the keto penne:

1 cup shredded mozzarella cheese
1 egg yolk

For the balsamic mix:

3 tbsp olive oil
1 medium red onion, thinly sliced
1 lb green beans, trimmed and halved
1 head broccoli, cut into florets
1 red bell pepper, deseeded and thinly sliced
5 garlic cloves, minced
Salt and black pepper to taste
1 tsp dried oregano
3 tbsp organic balsamic vinegar
1 cup grated Parmigiano-Reggiano cheese
2 tbsp chopped walnuts for topping

Directions

For the keto penne:

Pour the cheese into a medium safe-microwave bowl and melt in the microwave for 2 minutes while stirring at 20-second intervals until fully melted.

Take out the bowl and allow cooling for 1 minute only to warm the cheese but not cool completely. Mix in the egg yolk until well-combined.

Lay a parchment paper on a flat surface, pour the cheese mixture on top and cover with another parchment paper. Using a rolling pin, flatten the dough into 1/8-inch thickness.

Take off the parchment paper and cut the dough into mimicked penne-size pieces. Place in a bowl and refrigerate overnight. When ready to cook, bring 2 cups of water to a boil in medium saucepan and add the keto penne. Cook for 40 seconds to 1 minute and then drain through a colander. Run cold water over the pasta and set aside to cool.

For the balsamic mix:

Heat the olive oil in a large skillet and sauté the onion, green beans, broccoli, and bell pepper until softened, 5 to 7 minutes.

Stir in the garlic and cook until fragrant, 30 seconds, and season with salt, black pepper, and oregano.

Mix in the balsamic vinegar, cook for 1 minute and toss in the keto penne. Allow warming for 1 minute.

Adjust the taste with salt, black pepper and spoon the food onto serving plates.

Garnish with the Parmigiano-Reggiano cheese and walnuts.

Serve warm.

Nutritional info per serving:
Calories 326; Fats 21.2g; Net Carbs 7.5g; Protein 20g

Vegetarian Fajita Pasta

Mexican dishes are some of the most embraced ones around the world. I love that I can share this fajita mix with you.

Total Time: 20 minutes + chilling time| **Serving**: 4

Ingredients

For the keto penne:

1 cup shredded mozzarella cheese

1 egg yolk

For the fajita mix:

1 tsp olive oil

6 garlic cloves, minced

2 cups sugar-free enchilada sauce

1 tsp cumin powder

½ tsp smoked paprika

1 tsp chili powder

1 cup chopped mixed bell peppers

Salt and black pepper to taste

For topping:

¾ cup chopped green onions

1 large avocado, pitted, peeled and sliced

Directions

For the keto penne:

Pour the cheese into a medium safe-microwave bowl and melt in the microwave for 2 minutes while stirring at 20-second intervals. Take out the bowl and allow cooling for 1 minute only to warm the cheese but not cool completely. Mix in the egg yolk.

Lay a parchment paper on a flat surface, pour the cheese mixture on top and cover with another parchment paper. Using a rolling pin, flatten the dough into 1/8-inch thickness.

Take off the parchment paper and cut the dough into penne shapes. Refrigerate overnight. Bring 2 cups of water to a boil in saucepan and add the penne. Cook for 1 minute and then drain through a colander. Run cold water over the pasta and set aside to cool.

For the fajita mix:

Heat olive oil in a skillet and sauté garlic for 30 seconds. Mix in enchilada sauce, cumin powder, paprika, chili powder, bell peppers, salt, and pepper. Cook for 5 minutes. Add penne and mix well. Top with the green onions and avocado.

Nutritional info per serving:

Calories 151; Fats 7.9g; Net Carbs 3.3g; Protein 11.9g

Roasted Vegetable Spaghetti

Winter is here and making some pasta with roasted vegetables will be fantastic for the season.

Total Time: 45 minutes | **Serving**: 4

Ingredients

For the shirataki spaghetti:

2 (8 oz) packs shirataki spaghetti
Salt to season

For the roasted vegetable mix:

1 lb asparagus, trimmed and cut into ½-inch pieces
1 cup broccoli florets
1 cup chopped mixed bell peppers
1 cup green beans, trimmed and halved
3 tbsp olive oil
Salt and black pepper to taste
1 small onion, chopped
2 garlic cloves, minced
1 cup diced tomatoes
½ cup grated Parmesan cheese for topping
½ cup chopped fresh basil for garnishing

Directions

For the shirataki spaghetti:

Boil 2 cups of water in a medium pot over medium heat. Strain the shirataki pasta through a colander and rinse very well under hot running water. Allow proper draining and pour the shirataki pasta into the boiling water. Cook for 3 minutes and strain again.

Place a dry skillet over medium heat and stir-fry the shirataki pasta until visibly dry, and makes a squeaky sound when stirred, 1 to 2 minutes. Take off the heat and set aside.

For the roasted vegetable mix:

Preheat the oven to 425 F.

In a bowl, add asparagus, broccoli, bell peppers, green beans and toss with half of the olive oil, some salt and black pepper. Spread the vegetables on a baking sheet and roast in the oven until tender and slightly charred, 20 minutes. Meanwhile, occasionally mix.

Heat the remaining olive oil in a skillet and sauté onion and garlic for 3 minutes. Stir in tomatoes and cook for 8 minutes. Mix in shirataki spaghetti and roasted vegetables. Top with the Parmesan cheese and basil. Serve warm.

Nutritional info per serving:

Calories 272; Fats 11.5g; Net Carbs 20.9g; Protein 12.1g

Spicy Veggie Pasta Bake

Do you love chili? I do and surprisingly many keto dieters too. It takes away the fatigue of excessive creamy-cheesiness. This dish is one of my favorites.

Total Time: 45 minutes + overnight chilling time| **Serving**: 4

Ingredients

For the keto penne:

1 cup shredded mozzarella cheese
1 egg yolk

For the veggie bake:

1 tbsp olive oil
1 cup mixed chopped bell peppers
1 yellow squash, chopped
1 red onion, halved and sliced
1 cup sliced white button mushrooms
Salt and black pepper to taste
¼ tsp red chili flakes
1 cup sugar-free marinara sauce
1 cup grated mozzarella cheese
1 cup grated Parmesan cheese
¼ cup chopped fresh basil

Directions

For the keto penne:

Pour the cheese into a medium safe-microwave bowl and melt in the microwave for 2 minutes while stirring at 20-second intervals until fully melted.

Take out the bowl and allow cooling for 1 minute only to warm the cheese but not cool completely. Mix in the egg yolk until well-combined.

Lay a parchment paper on a flat surface, pour the cheese mixture on top and cover with another parchment paper. Using a rolling pin, flatten the dough into 1/8-inch thickness.

Take off the parchment paper and cut the dough into penne-size pieces. Place in a bowl and refrigerate overnight. When ready to cook, bring 2 cups of water to a boil in medium saucepan and add the keto penne. Cook for 40 seconds to 1 minute and then drain through a colander. Run cold water over the pasta and set aside to cool.

For the veggie bake:

Heat the olive oil in a large cast iron and sauté the bell peppers, squash, onion, and mushrooms. Cook until softened, 5 minutes. Stir in the garlic and cook until fragrant, 30 seconds. Season with the salt, black pepper, and red chili flakes.

Mix in the marinara sauce and cook for 5 minutes.

Stir in the keto penne and spread the mozzarella and Parmesan cheeses on top.

Bake in the oven until the cheeses melt and golden brown on top, 15 minutes.

Remove from the oven, allow cooling for 2 minutes and dish onto serving plates.

Serve warm.

Nutritional info per serving:
Calories 248; Fats 11.5g; Net Carbs 4.9g; Protein 26.8g

Super Green Pasta Skillet

Any health freaks out there? These green plates will set you in the right keto mood.

Total Time: 15 minutes + overnight chilling time| **Serving**: 4

Ingredients

For the keto fettuccine:

1 cup shredded mozzarella cheese

1 egg yolk

For the green sauce:

2 garlic cloves, minced

1 lemon, juiced

1 cup baby spinach

½ cup almond milk

1 small avocado, pitted and peeled

1 tbsp olive oil

Salt to taste

1 cup grated Pecorino Romano cheese

Directions

For the keto fettuccine:

Pour the cheese into a medium safe-microwave bowl and melt in the microwave for 2 minutes while stirring at 20-second intervals until fully melted.

Take out the bowl and allow cooling for 1 minute only to warm the cheese but not cool completely. Mix in the egg yolk until well-combined.

Lay a parchment paper on a flat surface, pour the cheese mixture on top and cover with another parchment paper. Using a rolling pin, flatten the dough into 1/8-inch thickness.

Take off the parchment paper and cut the dough into thick fettuccine strands. Place in a bowl and refrigerate overnight.

When ready to cook, bring 2 cups of water to a boil in medium saucepan and add the keto fettucine. Cook for 40 seconds to 1 minute and then drain through a colander. Run cold water over the pasta and set aside to cool.

For the green sauce:

In a blender, combine the garlic, lemon juice, spinach, almond milk, avocado, olive oil, and salt. Process until smooth. Pour the keto fettucine into a medium bowl, top with the sauce and mix well. Top with the Pecorino Romano cheese and serve warm.

Nutritional info per serving:

Calories 290; Fats 19.2g; Net Carbs 5.3g; Protein 18.2g

Broccoli and Pepper Spaghetti

An easy way to incorporate some veggies into your quick-fix pasta routine.

Total Time: 20 minutes | **Serving**: 4

Ingredients

2 tbsp olive oil
4 zucchinis, spiralized
1 head broccoli, cut into florets
1 cup sliced mixed bell peppers
4 shallots, finely chopped
Salt and black pepper to taste
2 garlic cloves, minced
¼ tsp red pepper flakes
1 cup chopped kale
2 tbsp organic balsamic vinegar
½ lemon, juiced
1 cup grated Parmesan cheese

Directions

Heat the olive oil in a large skillet and sauté the turnips, broccoli, bell peppers, and shallots until softened, 7 minutes. Mix in the garlic, red pepper flakes and cook until fragrant, 30 seconds.

Stir in the kale and zucchinis; cook until tender, 2 to 3 minutes.

Mix in the vinegar, lemon juice and adjust the taste with salt and black pepper.

Dish the food onto serving plates and garnish with the Parmesan cheese.

Serve warm.

Nutritional info per serving:

Calories 199; Fats 13.9g; Net Carbs 5.9g; Protein 8.8g

Veggie Pasta Primavera

Even better to incorporate some tang and Italian flavors into a simple veggie-pasta blend.

Total Time: 25 minutes + overnight chilling time| **Serving**: 4

Ingredients

For the keto penne:

1 cup shredded mozzarella cheese

1 egg yolk

For the veggie mix:

¼ cup olive oil

½ cup chopped fresh green (spring) onions

2 cups cauliflower florets, cut into matchsticks

1 red bell pepper, deseeded and thinly sliced

4 garlic cloves, minced

1 cup grape tomatoes, halved

2 tsp dried Italian seasoning

½ lemon, juiced

½ cup grated Pecorino Romano cheese

2 tbsp chopped fresh parsley

Directions

For the keto penne:

Pour the cheese into a medium safe-microwave bowl and melt in the microwave for 2 minutes while stirring at 20-second intervals until fully melted. Take out the bowl and allow cooling for 1 minute only to warm the cheese but not cool completely. Mix in the egg yolk until well-combined.

Lay a parchment paper on a flat surface, pour the cheese mixture on top and cover with another parchment paper. Using a rolling pin, flatten the dough into 1/8-inch thickness. Take off the parchment paper and cut the dough into penne-size pieces. Place in a bowl and refrigerate overnight. Bring 2 cups of water to a boil in saucepan and add the keto penne. Cook for 1 minute and then drain. Set aside to cool.

For the veggie mix:

Heat olive oil in a skillet and sauté onion, cauliflower, and bell pepper for 7 minutes. Mix in garlic and cook until fragrant, 30 seconds. Stir in the tomatoes and Italian seasoning; cook until the tomatoes soften, 5 minutes. Mix in the lemon juice, keto penne and adjust the taste with salt and black pepper. Garnish with the Pecorino Romano cheese.

Nutritional info per serving:

Calories 283; Fats 18.5g; Net Carbs 5.2g; Protein 15.2g

PIZZA

Pepperoni Fat Head Pizza

My favorite pizza had to be first! The terrific taste is in the crust.

Total Time: 35 minutes | **Serving**: 4

Ingredients
1 ½ cups + 2 cups grated mozzarella cheese
2 tbsp cream cheese, room temperature
2 eggs, beaten
1/3 cup almond flour
1 tsp dried oregano
½ cup sliced pepperoni

Directions
Preheat the oven to 425 F and line a round pizza pan with parchment paper.

Combine 1 ½ cups of the mozzarella cheese and cream cheese in a safe-microwave bowl and melt in the microwave for 1 minute.

Remove from the oven and mix in the eggs and almond flour. Transfer the mixture onto a clean flat surface and knead until smooth.

Spread the dough on the pizza pan and bake in the oven for 6 minutes or until golden brown and crusty.

Remove from the oven, top with the remaining mozzarella cheese, oregano, and pepperoni slices.

Bake further in the oven for 15 minutes or until the cheese melts.

Remove the pizza, slice and serve.

Nutritional info per serving:
Calories 229; Fats 7.1g; Net Carbs 0.4g; Protein 36.4g

BBQ Beef Pizza

Likewise, beef makes the crust weighty and satisfying. Meanwhile, the pizza itself offers excellent BBQ aromas.

Total Time: 40 minutes | **Serving**: 4

Ingredients

For the crust:

1 lb ground beef
1 cup grated mozzarella cheese
2 eggs, beaten
¼ tsp salt

For topping:

¼ cup sugar-free BBQ sauce
1 ½ cups grated Gruyere cheese
¼ cup sliced red onion
2 bacon slices, chopped
2 tbsp chopped parsley

Directions

Preheat the oven to 425 F and line a pizza pan with parchment paper.

In a medium bowl, mix the beef, mozzarella cheese, eggs, and salt.

Spread the mixture on the pizza pan and bake in the oven for 20 minutes or until the meat cooks and is crusty.

Remove the crust from the oven and spread the BBQ sauce on top. Scatter the Gruyere cheese on top, followed by the red onion, and bacon slices.

Bake in the oven for 15 minutes or until the cheese has melted and the back is crispy.

Remove the pizza from the oven, slice and serve warm sprinkled with parsley.

Nutritional info per serving:

Calories 538; Fats 32.9g; Net Carbs 0.4g; Protein 55.8g

Chicken-Basil Pizza

A more enjoyable crust with chicken serving as the base of the crust and pizza.

Total Time: 40 minutes | **Serving**: 4

Ingredients

For the crust:

1 lb ground chicken
1 tsp Italian seasoning
½ cup grated mozzarella cheese
¼ tsp salt

For the topping:

⅔ cup sugar-free tomato sauce
1 cup grated mozzarella cheese
½ cup fresh basil leaves

Directions

Preheat the oven to 425 F and line a pizza pan with parchment paper.

In a medium bowl, mix the ground chicken, Italian seasoning, mozzarella cheese, and salt until well combined.

Spread the mixture on the pizza pan and bake in the oven until the chicken is cooked and crusty, 18 minutes.

Remove from the oven and spread the tomato sauce on top. Scatter the mozzarella cheese on top and then the basil.

Bake further for 15 minutes or until the cheese melts.

Remove from the oven, slice and serve warm.

Nutritional info per serving:

Calories 316; Fats 17.2g; Net Carbs 0.4g; Protein 35g

Chicken Bacon Ranch Pizza

Ranch seasoning is right for salads, casseroles as well as this pizza. And it always works perfectly with chicken.

Total Time: 45 minutes | **Serving**: 4

Ingredients

For the crust:

2 cups shredded mozzarella cheese
2 tbsp cream cheese
¾ cup almond flour
2 tbsp almond meal

For the ranch sauce:

1 tbsp butter
2 garlic cloves, minced
1 tbsp cream cheese
¼ cup half and half
1 tbsp dry Ranch seasoning mix

For the topping:

3 bacon slices, chopped
2 chicken breasts
Salt and black pepper to taste
1 cup grated mozzarella cheese
6 fresh basil leaves

Directions

Preheat the oven to 425 F and line a pizza pan with parchment paper.

In a safe-microwave bowl, combine the mozzarella and cream cheese. Melt in the microwave for 1 minute. Remove the bowl from the oven and mix in the almond flour and almond meal. Spread the mixture on the pizza pan and bake for 15 minutes.

Meanwhile, in a medium, mix the sauce's ingredients butter, garlic, cream cheese, half and half, and ranch mix. Set aside.

Heat a grill pan over medium heat and cook the bacon until crispy and brown, 5 minutes. Transfer to a plate and set aside.

Season the chicken with salt, pepper and grill in the pan on both sides until golden brown, 10 minutes. Remove to a plate, allow cooling and cut into thin slices. Spread the ranch sauce on the pizza crust, followed by the chicken and bacon, and then, mozzarella cheese and basil. Bake for 5 minutes or until the cheese melts. Slice and serve warm.

Nutritional info per serving:

Calories 528; Fats 27.8g; Net Carbs 4.9g; Protein 61.2g

Kale-Artichoke Pizza

This pizza screams excellent health with a luscious topping of creamed greens.

Total Time: 45 minutes | **Serving**: 4

Ingredients

For the crust:

1 ½ cups grated mozzarella cheese
2 tbsp cream cheese
1 egg, beaten
1 tsp Italian seasoning
½ tsp garlic powder
½ cup almond flour

For the topping:

4 tbsp cream cheese, room temperature
½ cup chopped kale
¼ cup chopped artichoke
1 lemon, juiced
½ tsp garlic powder
¼ cup grated Parmesan cheese
½ cup grated Mozzarella cheese
Salt and black pepper to taste

Directions

Preheat the oven to 425 F and line a pizza pan with parchment paper.

In a medium safe-microwave bowl, combine the mozzarella and cream cheese. Melt in the microwave for 30 seconds to 1 minute. Remove the bowl from the oven and mix in the egg, Italian seasoning, garlic powder, and almond flour. Spread the mixture on the pizza pan and bake in the oven for 15 minutes or until crusty. Remove the crust from the oven and set aside to cool.

In a medium bowl, mix the cream cheese, kale, artichoke, lemon juice, garlic powder, Parmesan cheese, mozzarella cheese, salt, and black pepper. Spread the mixture on the crust and bake again for 15 minutes or slightly golden.

Nutritional info per serving:

Calories 223; Fats 10.7g; Net Carbs 3.1g; Protein 24.4g

Sausage-Pepper Pizza

Mixed bell peppers offer sweet aromas to this pizza as a compliment to the intense flavor of Italian sausages.

Total Time: 45 minutes | **Serving**: 4

Ingredients

For the crust:

1 ½ cups grated mozzarella cheese
2 tbsp cream cheese, room temperature
1 ½ lb Italian sausages, crumbled
¼ cup coconut flour
1 cup almond flour
¼ cup grated Parmesan cheese
2 eggs

For the topping:

1 tbsp olive oil
1 onion, thinly sliced
1 cup chopped mixed bell peppers
2 garlic cloves, minced
1 cup baby spinach
½ cup sugar-free pizza sauce
2 cups grated mozzarella cheese
½ cup grated Monterey Jack cheese

Directions

Preheat the oven to 425 F and line a pizza pan with parchment paper.

In a medium safe-microwave bowl, combine the mozzarella and cream cheese. Melt in the microwave for 30 seconds to 1 minute.

Remove the bowl from the oven and mix in the sausages, coconut flour, almond flour, Parmesan cheese, and eggs. Spread the mixture on the pizza pan and bake in the oven for 15 minutes or until crusty. Remove from the oven and set aside to cool for 2 minutes.

Meanwhile, heat the olive oil in a medium skillet and sauté the onion and bell peppers until softened, 5 minutes. Mix in the garlic and cook until fragrant, 30 seconds. Stir in the spinach and allow wilting for 3 minutes. Turn the heat off.

Spread the pizza sauce on the crust and top with the bell pepper mixture. Scatter the mozzarella and Monterey Jack cheeses on top.

Bake in the oven for 5 minutes or until the cheese melts. Remove from the oven, slice, and serve warm.

Nutritional info per serving:

Calories 460; Fats 25.6g; Net Carbs 3.2g; Protein 46.7g

Tomato-Prosciutto Pizza

What would have been a regular tomato pizza turns out to be more delicious with a draping of prosciutto slices.

Total Time: 45 minutes | **Serving**: 4

Ingredients

For the crust:

1 ½ cups grated mozzarella cheese
2 tbsp cream cheese
½ cup almond meal
1 egg, beaten

For the topping:

⅓ cup sugar-free tomato sauce
⅓ cup sliced mozzarella
4 prosciutto slices, cut into thirds
7 fresh basil leaves, to serve

Directions

Preheat the oven to 425 F and line a pizza pan with parchment paper.

In a medium safe-microwave bowl, combine the mozzarella and cream cheese. Melt in the microwave for 30 seconds to 1 minute.

Remove the bowl from the oven and mix in the almond meal and egg.

Spread the mixture on the pizza pan and bake in the oven for 15 minutes or until crusty.

Remove the crust from the oven and set aside to cool.

Spread the tomato sauce on the crust. Arrange the mozzarella slices on the sauce and then the prosciutto.

Bake again for 15 minutes or until the cheese melts.

Remove from the oven and top with the basil. Slice and serve warm.

Nutritional info per serving:

Calories 160; Fats 6.2g; Net Carbs 0.5g; Protein 21.9g

Vegetarian Spinach-Olive Pizza

A tasty, quickly-satisfying option for vegetarians.

Total Time: 40 minutes | **Serving**: 4

Ingredients

For the crust:

½ cup almond flour
¼ tsp salt
2 tbsp ground psyllium husk
1 tbsp olive oil
1 cup lukewarm water

For the topping:

½ cup sugar-free tomato sauce
½ cup baby spinach
1 cup grated mozzarella cheese
1 tsp dried oregano
3 tbsp sliced black olives

Directions

Preheat the oven to 425 F and line a baking sheet with parchment paper.

In a medium bowl, mix the almond flour, salt, psyllium powder, olive oil, and water until dough forms.

Spread the mixture on the pizza pan and bake in the oven until crusty, 10 minutes.

When ready, remove the crust and spread the tomato sauce on top.

Add the spinach, mozzarella cheese, oregano, and olives.

Bake until the cheese melts, 15 minutes.

Take out of the oven, slice and serve warm.

Nutritional info per serving:

Calories 95; Fats 4.3g; Net Carbs 1.8g; Protein 9.7g

Cauliflower-Pepperoni Pizza Casserole

The right way to make the best cauliflower crust is to include a generous amount of mozzarella cheese. And that's what I rock here! You'll love it!

Total Time: 40 minutes | **Serving**: 4

Ingredients

4 cups cauliflower rice
1 cup grated mozzarella cheese
1 tbsp dried thyme
Salt and black pepper to taste

For the topping:

¼ cup sugar-free tomato sauce
1 cup grated mozzarella cheese
½ cup pepperoni slices

Directions

Preheat the oven to 425 F and lightly grease a baking dish with cooking spray. Set aside.

Pour the cauliflower rice in a safe microwave bowl, mix in 1 tablespoon of water and steam in the microwave for 1 minute.

Remove the bowl and mix in the mozzarella cheese, thyme, salt, and black pepper. Pour the mixture into the baking dish, spread out and bake in the oven for 5 minutes.

Take the dish out of the oven and spread the tomato sauce on top. Scatter the mozzarella cheese on the sauce and then arrange the pepperoni slices on top.

Bake in the oven for 15 more minutes or until the cheese melts.

Remove the dish and serve the pizza casserole warm.

Nutritional info per serving:

Calories 116; Fats 0.4g; Net Carbs 1.7g; Protein 20.4g

Italian Mushroom Pizza

Burger ideas and pizzas unite in this offering. Enjoy the kick and moreish tastes.

Total Time: 45 minutes | **Serving**: 4

Ingredients

For the crust:

1 ½ cups grated mozzarella cheese
2 tbsp cream cheese
½ cup almond meal
1 egg, beaten

For the topping:

1 tsp olive oil
2 medium cremini mushrooms, sliced
1 garlic clove, minced
½ cup sugar-free tomato sauce
1 tsp erythritol
1 bay leaf
1 tsp dried oregano
1 tsp dried basil
1/2 tsp paprika
Salt and black pepper to taste
½ cup grated mozzarella cheese
½ cup grated Parmesan cheese
6 black olives, pitted and sliced

Directions

Preheat the oven to 425 F and line a pizza pan with parchment paper.

In a medium safe-microwave bowl, combine the mozzarella and cream cheese. Melt in the microwave for 30 seconds to 1 minute. Remove the bowl from the oven and mix in the almond meal and egg. Spread the mixture on the pizza pan and bake in the oven for 5 minutes or until crusty. Remove the crust from the oven and set aside to cool.

Meanwhile, heat the olive oil in a medium skillet and sauté the mushrooms until softened, 5 minutes. Stir in the garlic and cook until fragrant, 30 seconds.

Mix in the tomato sauce, erythritol, bay leaf, oregano, basil, paprika, salt, and black pepper. Cook for 2 minutes and turn the heat off.

Spread the sauce on the crust, top with the mozzarella and Parmesan cheeses, and then, the olives.

Bake in the oven until the cheeses melts, 15 minutes.

Remove the pizza, slice and serve warm.

Nutritional info per serving:

Calories 203; Fats 8.6g; Net Carbs 2.6g; Protein 24.3g

Extra Cheesy Pizza

Are you feeling extra? Work in plenty of cheeses, don't be limited with your cheese choices.

Total Time: 35 minutes | **Serving**: 4

Ingredients

For the crust:

½ cup almond flour
¼ tsp salt
2 tbsp ground psyllium husk
1 tbsp olive oil
1 cup lukewarm water

For the topping:

½ cup sugar-free pizza sauce
1 cup sliced mozzarella cheese
1 cup grated mozzarella cheese
3 tbsp grated Parmesan cheese
2 tsp Italian seasoning

Directions

Preheat the oven to 425 F and line a baking sheet with parchment paper.

In a medium bowl, mix the almond flour, salt, psyllium powder, olive oil, and lukewarm water until dough forms.

Spread the mixture on the pizza pan and bake in the oven until crusty, 10 minutes.

When ready, remove the crust and spread the pizza sauce on top. Add the sliced mozzarella, grated mozzarella, Parmesan cheese, and Italian seasoning.

Bake in the oven for 18 minutes or until the cheeses melt.

Remove from the oven, slice and serve warm.

Nutritional info per serving:

Calories 193; Fats 10.2g; Net Carbs 3.2g; Protein 19.5g

Spicy and Smoky Pizza

Two worlds combine on a pizza crust! There's so much enjoyment to derive.

Total Time: 45 minutes | **Serving**: 4

Ingredients

For the crust:

2 cups shredded mozzarella cheese
2 tbsp cream cheese
¾ cup almond flour
2 tbsp almond meal

For the topping:

1 tbsp olive oil
1 cups sliced chorizo
¼ cup sugar-free marinara sauce
1 cup sliced smoked mozzarella cheese
1 jalapeño pepper, deseeded and sliced
¼ red onion, thinly sliced

Directions

Preheat the oven to 425 F and line a pizza pan with parchment paper.

In a medium safe-microwave bowl, combine the mozzarella and cream cheese. Melt in the microwave for 30 seconds to 1 minute.

Remove the bowl from the oven and mix in the almond flour and almond meal.

Spread the mixture on the pizza pan and bake in the oven for 10 minutes or until crusty.

Remove the crust from the oven and set aside to cool.

Meanwhile, heat the olive oil and cook the chorizo until brown, 5 minutes.

Spread the marinara sauce on the crust, top with the mozzarella cheese, chorizo, jalapeño pepper, and onion.

Bake in the oven until the cheese melts, 15 minutes.

Remove from the oven, slice and serve warm.

Nutritional info per serving:

Calories 302; Fats 17g; Net Carbs 1.4g; Protein 31.6g

Taco pizza

Not up for dripping taco juices on your shirt? Combine all the ingredients into this pizza and enjoy the ease.

Total Time: 45 minutes | **Serving**: 4

Ingredients

For the crust:

2 cups shredded mozzarella
2 tbsp cream cheese
1 egg
¾ cup almond flour

For the topping:

1 lb ground beef
2 tsp taco seasoning
Salt and black pepper to taste
½ cup cheese sauce
1 cup grated cheddar cheese
1 cup chopped lettuce
1 tomato, diced
¼ cup sliced black olives
1 cup sour cream for topping

Directions

Preheat the oven to 425 F and line a pizza pan with parchment paper.

In a medium safe-microwave bowl, combine the mozzarella and cream cheese. Melt in the microwave for 30 seconds to 1 minute. Remove the bowl from the oven and mix in the egg and almond flour. Spread the mixture on the pizza pan and bake in the oven for 15 minutes or until crusty. Remove the crust from the oven and set aside to cool.

Meanwhile, put the beef in a pot and cook until brown, 5 minutes. Stir in taco seasoning, salt, and pepper. Spread the cheese sauce on the crust and top with the meat. Add the cheddar cheese, lettuce, tomato, and black olives. Bake until the cheese melts, 5 minutes. Remove the pizza from the oven, drizzle the sour cream on top, slice, and serve warm.

Nutritional info per serving:

Calories 590; Fats 29g; Net Carbs 8g; Protein 64g

Broccoli-Pepper Pizza

It is loaded, quickly-filling and juicy. Broccoli and peppers make for the best couple on this low-carb crust.

Total Time: 25 minutes | **Serving**: 4

Ingredients

For the crust:

½ cup almond flour
¼ tsp salt
2 tbsp ground psyllium husk
1 tbsp olive oil
1 cup lukewarm water

For the topping:

1 tbsp olive oil
1 cup sliced fresh mushrooms
1 white onion, thinly sliced
3 cups broccoli florets
4 garlic cloves, minced
½ cup sugar-free pizza sauce
4 tomatoes, sliced
¼ cup chopped basil
1 ½ cup grated mozzarella cheese
⅓ cup grated Parmesan cheese

Directions

Preheat the oven to 425 F and line a baking sheet with parchment paper.

In a bowl, mix the almond flour, salt, psyllium powder, olive oil, and lukewarm water until dough forms. Spread the mixture on the pizza pan and bake in the oven until crusty, 10 minutes. When ready, remove the crust and allow cooling.

Heat olive oil in a skillet and sauté the mushrooms, onion, garlic, and broccoli until softened, 5 minutes. Spread the pizza sauce on the crust and top with the broccoli mixture, tomato, basil, mozzarella and Parmesan cheeses. Bake for 5 minutes. Serve.

Nutritional info per serving:

Calories 180; Fats 9g; Net Carbs 3.6g; Protein 17g

Caramelized Onion and Goat Cheese Pizza

A mimicked French onion soup blend. Instead, I find goat cheese to offer a better flavor than Gruyere cheese in this case.

Total Time: 35 minutes | **Serving**: 4

Ingredients

For the crust:
2 cups grated mozzarella cheese
2 tbsp cream cheese, room temperature
2 large eggs, beaten
⅓ cup almond flour
1 tsp dried Italian seasoning

For the topping:

2 tbsp butter
2 red onions, thinly sliced
Salt and black pepper to taste
1 cup crumbled goat cheese
1 tbs almond milk
1 cup fresh curly endive, chopped

Directions

Preheat the oven to 425 F and line a round pizza pan with parchment paper.

Combine the mozzarella cheese and cream cheese in a safe-microwave bowl and melt in the microwave for 1 minute. Remove from the oven and mix in the eggs, almond flour, and Italian seasoning. Spread the dough on the pizza pan and bake in the oven for 6 minutes or until golden brown and crusty.

Meanwhile, melt the butter in a large skillet and stir in the onions. Reduce the heat to low, season the onions with salt, black pepper, and cook with frequent stirring until caramelized, 15 to 20 minutes. Turn the heat.

In a medium bowl, mix the goat cheese with the almond milk and spread on the crust. Top with the caramelized onions. Bake in the oven for 10 minutes and take out after. Top with the curly endive, slice the pizza and serve warm.

Nutritional info per serving:

Calories 317; Fats 20g; Net Carbs 1g; Protein 28g

Shrimp Scampi Pizza

A fantastic way to incorporate shrimp into your pizza-making. This topping is a full-fledged meal in itself. Serve this for lunch and dinner, and you'll still want to enjoy some leftovers for breakfast.

Total Time: 35 minutes | **Serving**: 4

Ingredients

For the crust:

½ cup almond flour
¼ tsp salt
2 tbsp ground psyllium husk
1 tbsp olive oil
1 cup lukewarm water

For the topping:

2 tbsp butter
2 tbsp olive oil
2 garlic cloves, minced
¼ cup white wine
½ tsp dried basil
½ tsp dried parsley
½ lemon, juiced
½ lb medium shrimp, peeled and deveined
2 cups grated cheese blend
½ tsp Italian seasoning
¼ cup grated Parmesan cheese

Directions

Preheat the oven to 425 F and line a baking sheet with parchment paper.

In a medium bowl, mix the almond flour, salt, psyllium powder, olive oil, and lukewarm water until dough forms. Spread the mixture on the pizza pan and bake in the oven until crusty, 10 minutes. When ready, remove the crust and allow cooling.

Meanwhile, heat the butter and olive oil in a medium skillet. Sauté the garlic until fragrant, 30 seconds. Mix in the white wine, allow reduction by half and stir in the basil, parsley, and lemon juice. Cook for 1 minute and stir in the shrimp. Cook for 3 minutes or until pink and opaque. Stir in the cheese blend and Italian seasoning. Allow cheese melting, 3 minutes. Turn the heat off.

Spread the shrimp mixture on the crust and top with the Parmesan cheese. Bake for 5 minutes or until the Parmesan cheese has melted. Remove the pizza from the oven, slice and serve warm.

Nutritional info per serving:

Calories 423; Fats 34g; Net Carbs 4g; Protein 23g

Strawberry-Tomato Pizza

A fruity mix for when you want something sweet.

Total Time: 35 minutes | **Serving**: 4

Ingredients

For the crust:

2 cups shredded mozzarella cheese
2 tbsp cream cheese
¾ cup almond flour
2 tbsp almond meal

For the topping:

1 cup grated mozzarella cheese
2 celery stalks, chopped
1 medium tomato, chopped
1 tbsp olive oil
Salt and black pepper to taste
2 tbsp balsamic vinegar, divided
1 cup fresh strawberries, halved
1 tbsp chopped mint leaves

Directions

Preheat the oven to 425 F and line a pizza pan with parchment paper.

In a medium safe-microwave bowl, combine the mozzarella and cream cheese. Melt in the microwave for 30 seconds to 1 minute. Remove the bowl from the oven and mix in the almond flour and almond meal. Spread the mixture on the pizza pan and bake in the oven for 10 minutes or until crusty. Remove the crust from the oven and set aside to cool. Spread the mozzarella cheese on the crust.

In a medium bowl, toss the celery and tomato with the olive oil, salt, black pepper, and balsamic vinegar. Spoon the mixture onto the mozzarella cheese and arrange the strawberries on top. Top with the mint leaves. Bake in the oven until the cheese melts, 15 minutes. Remove the pizza from the oven, slice and serve warm.

Nutritional info per serving:

Calories 206; Fats 6g; Net Carbs 1g; Protein 28g

Mediterranean Pizza

A given for the love of healthy foods and one from the Mediterranean coast.

Total Time: 30 minutes | **Serving**: 4

Ingredients

For the crust:

½ cup almond flour
¼ tsp salt
2 tbsp ground psyllium husk
1 tbsp olive oil
1 cup lukewarm water

For the topping:

¼ tsp red chili flakes
¼ tsp dried Italian seasoning
1 cup crumbled feta cheese
3 sliced plum tomatoes
6 pitted Kalamata olives, chopped
5 basil leaves, chopped for garnishing

Directions

Preheat the oven to 425 F and line a baking sheet with parchment paper.

In a medium bowl, mix the almond flour, salt, psyllium powder, olive oil, and lukewarm water until dough forms.

Spread the mixture on the pizza pan and bake in the oven until crusty, 10 minutes.

When ready, remove the crust and allow cooling.

Sprinkle the red chili flakes and Italian seasoning on the crust and top with the feta cheese.

Use the back of a spoon to press the cheese onto the crust and arrange the tomatoes and olives on top.

Bake in the oven for 10 to 12 minutes and remove afterwards.

Garnish the pizza with the basil, slice and serve warm.

Nutritional info per serving:

Calories 176; Fats 12g; Net Carbs 1.5g; Protein 5.8g

Pesto Arugula Pizza

Easy, breezy and bursting with the smell of fresh vegetables!

Total Time: 30 minutes | **Serving**: 4

Ingredients

For the crust:

½ cup almond flour
¼ tsp salt
2 tbsp ground psyllium husk
1 tbsp olive oil
1 cup lukewarm water

For the topping:

1 cup basil pesto, olive oil-based
1 cup grated mozzarella cheese
1 tomato, thinly sliced
1 zucchini, cut into half-moon pieces
1 cup baby arugula
2 tbsp chopped pecans
¼ tsp red chili flakes

Directions

Preheat the oven to 425 F and line a baking sheet with parchment paper.

In a medium bowl, mix the almond flour, salt, psyllium powder, olive oil, and lukewarm water until dough forms.

Spread the mixture on the pizza pan and bake in the oven until crusty, 10 minutes.

When ready, remove the crust and allow cooling.

Spread the pesto on the crust and top with the mozzarella cheese, tomato, and zucchini.

Bake in the oven until the cheese melts, 15 minutes.

Remove the pizza from the oven; top with the arugula, pecans, and red chili flakes.

Slice and serve the pizza warm.

Nutritional info per serving:

Calories 186; Fats 14g; Net Carbs 1.4g; Protein 11g

Four Cheese Mexican Pizza

Grab your four favorite Mexican cheeses, place them on a pizza crust and bake away!

Total Time: 50 minutes | **Serving**: 4

Ingredients

For the crust:

2 cups shredded mozzarella cheese
2 tbsp cream cheese
¾ cup almond flour
2 eggs, beaten

For the topping:

¾ lb ground beef
2 tsp taco seasoning mix
Salt and black pepper to taste
½ cup chicken broth
1 ½ cups salsa
2 cups Mexican four cheese blend

Directions

Preheat the oven to 425 F and line a pizza pan with parchment paper.

In a medium safe-microwave bowl, combine the mozzarella and cream cheese. Melt in the microwave for 30 seconds to 1 minute.

Remove the bowl from the oven and mix in the almond flour and eggs.

Spread the mixture on the pizza pan and bake in the oven for 15 minutes or until crusty.

Remove the crust from the oven and set aside to cool.

Add the beef to a medium pot and cook until brown, 5 minutes. Stir in the taco seasoning, salt, black pepper and chicken broth. Cook for 3 minutes or until thickened. Stir in the salsa. Spread the beef mixture onto the crust and scatter the cheese blend on top.

Bake further in the oven until the cheese melts, 15 minutes.

Remove the pizza, slice and serve warm

Nutritional info per serving:

Calories 556; Fats 30g; Net Carbs 2g; Protein 59g

SOMETHING SWEET

Italian Raspberry-Coconut Cake

A no-fuss cake with lots of creaminess and fruitiness. Healthy and sweet to be enjoyed day-long.

Total Time: 30 minutes + chilling time| **Serving**: 6

Ingredients

2 cups flaxseed meal
1 cup almond meal
½ cup melted butter
2 cups fresh raspberries, mashed + extra for topping
1 lemon, juiced
1 cup coconut cream
1 cup unsweetened coconut flakes
1 cup whipping cream

Directions

Preheat the oven to 400 F.

In a medium bowl, mix the flaxseed meal, almond meal, and butter. Spread the mixture in the bottom of a small baking dish. Bake in the oven for 20 minutes until the mixture is crusty.

Remove the dish from the oven and allow cooling.

In another bowl, mix the raspberries with the lemon juice. Spread the mixture on the crust.

Carefully, spread the coconut cream on top, scatter with the coconut flakes and add the whipped cream all over.

Garnish with 10 to 12 raspberries and chill in the refrigerator for at least 2 hours.

Serve afterwards.

Nutritional info per serving:

Calories 556; Fats 55g; Net Carbs 10g; Protein 32g

Balsamic Strawberry Ricotta

Alternately, layer your favorite keto fruit with ricotta cheese on a dessert plate. Add some tang and sweetness, and enjoy. That simple!

Total Time: 10 minutes | **Serving**: 4

Ingredients
2 cups fresh strawberries, chopped
1 cup ricotta cheese
2 tbsp sugar-free maple syrup
2 tbsp balsamic vinegar

Directions
Divide half of the strawberries onto 4 dessert plates and top with the ricotta cheese.

Drizzle with the maple syrup, balsamic vinegar and top with the remaining strawberries.

Serve immediately.

Nutritional info per serving:
Calories 164; Fats 8g; Net Carbs 8g; Protein 7g

Blueberry Sorbet

Since we can't have regular ice cream on the keto diet, we will have some sorbet instead! And this one rocks!

Total Time: 15 minutes + 6 hours chilling | **Serving**: 4

Ingredients
4 cups frozen blueberries
1 cup swerve sugar
½ lemon, juiced
½ tsp salt

Directions
In a blender, add the blueberries, swerve sugar, lemon juice, and salt. Process until smooth. Strain the mixture through a colander into a bowl. Chill for 2 to 3 hours.

Pour the chilled juice into an ice cream maker and churn until the mixture resembles ice cream.

Spoon into a bowl and chill further for 3 hours.

Serve when ready to enjoy.

Nutritional info per serving:
Calories 178; Fats 1g; Net Carbs 2.3g; Protein 1g

Strawberry Mousse

I saved one of the bests for the last and it is my favorite dessert-in-a-glass recipes. You can swap the berries based on your preference and it will turn out fantastic too.

Total Time: 10 minutes + 2 hours chilling | **Serving**: 4

Ingredients
2 ½ cups frozen strawberries + more for garnishing
2 tbsp swerve sugar
1 large egg white
2 cups whipped cream

Directions
Pour the strawberries into a blender and process until smooth.

Add the swerve sugar and process further. Pour in the egg white and blend until well combined.

Pour the mixture into a medium bowl and use an electric hand mixer to whisk until fluffy.

Spoon the mixture into dessert glasses, top with the whipped cream and then, some strawberries.

Chill for 2 hours and serve afterwards.

Nutritional info per serving:
Calories 145; Fats 7g; Net Carbs 4.8g; Protein 2g

Sweet Lemon Panna Cotta

Talk of the Italian cuisine and panna cotta has to be involved. Here is my favorite one.

Total Time: 30 minutes + 7 hours chilling | **Serving**: 4

Ingredients

½ cup coconut milk
1 cup heavy cream
¼ cup swerve sugar
5 tbsp sugar-free maple syrup
3 tsp agar agar
¼ cup warm water
3 tbsp water
½ lemon, juiced

Directions

Heat the coconut milk and heavy cream in a medium pot over low heat.

Stir in the swerve sugar, 3 tablespoons of the maple syrup, and 2 teaspoons of the agar agar. Continue cooking for 2 to 3 minutes. Cool completely and divide the mixture into 4 dessert cups. Chill in the refrigerator for 5 hours or until set.

In a medium bowl, soak the remaining agar agar with the warm water. Allow blooming for 5 minutes.

In a small pot, heat 3 tbsp of water with the lemon juice. Mix in the remaining maple syrup and add the agar mixture. Continually whisking while cooking until no lumps form.

Turn the heat off and cool for 2 minutes.

Remove the dessert cups, pour in the mixture and refrigerate further for 2 hours.

When ready to serve, take out the cups, allow sitting for 15 minutes and then enjoy afterwards.

Nutritional info per serving:

Calories 208; Fats 18g; Net Carbs 2.8g; Protein 2g

Made in the USA
Coppell, TX
13 March 2020